Passing Medical Examinations

A handbook for final qualifying and postgraduate
examinations and for all their examiners

Second edition

M. H. Pappworth, MD, MRCP

Butterworths
London Boston Durban Singapore Sydney Toronto Wellington

First published, 1975
Reprinted 1975
Reprinted 1978
Reprinted 1980
Second edition, 1985

© **Butterworth & Co. (Publishers) Ltd, 1985**

British Library Cataloguing in Publication Data

Pappworth, M.H.
  Passing medical examinations: a handbook for
  final qualifying and postgraduate examinations
  and for all their examiners.–2nd ed.
  1. Medical personnel–Examinations, questions,
  etc. 2. Medical education–Great Britain
  I. Title
  610′.76   R772

  ISBN 0-407-00415-7

Library of Congress Cataloging in Publication Data

Pappworth, M.H. (Maurice Henry)
  Passing medical examinations.

  Includes index.
  1. Medicine–Examinations. 2. Medicine–Great
  Britain–Examinations. I. Title. [DNLM: 1. Educational
  Measurement. WY 18 P218p]
  R834.5.P36 1985   610′.76   85-7783
  ISBN 0-407-00415-7

Photoset by Butterworths Litho Preparation Department
Printed in England by Page Bros Ltd., Norwich, Norfolk

Passing Medical Examinations

This book is dedicated to my daughters Joanna, Dinah, and Sarah, wishing them in the words from the Benediction proclaiming the forthcoming New Moon (Jewish Calendar Month):

'A long life; a life of peace, of good, of blessing, of sustenance, of bodily vigour; a life marked by reverence for Heaven and awareness of the consequences of sin; a life free from shame and reproach; a life of prosperity and honour.'

By the same author
A Primer of Medicine (5th edition 1984)
Human Guinea Pigs

Preface

'It is always silly to give advice but to give good advice is absolutely fatal.'

I hope that this quip of Oscar Wilde does not apply to this book.

In 1972 I was asked to lecture at each of several Eire and Belfast (Northern Ireland) medical schools. Different subjects had been suggested to me by each medical school. But I felt unable to accept all the invitations and urged them to combine and arrange a joint meeting, preferably at University College, Dublin, because they had been the first to approach me. This was finally agreed.

The lecture was considered to have been a great success. Over 400 attended; and, most important, probably for the first time in their long history, University College (a Catholic foundation) combined with Trinity College, Dublin (a Protestant foundation) in a joint meeting. Students also come from the Royal College of Surgeons (Dublin) and Galway Medical School, and, most exciting of all, over 40 came especially from Belfast. So, I, a non-Christian, united Catholics and Protestants if only for one night. I shall always regard this as one of the highlights of my long career. This book is based on that, to me, memorable lecture.

That meeting reinforced my belief that it is incumbent on everybody, whatever their religious belief or even if they are totally irreligious, to strive to establish the brotherhood of man, a principle which cannot be reconciled with racial or sectarian quarrels.

'Behold, how good and how pleasant it is for brethren to dwell together in unity.'

Psalm 133, verse 1.

'Have not all one Father? Did not one God create us?'

Malachi 2:10.

'Be kindly and affectionate one to another with brotherly love.'
St. Paul's Epistle to the Romans 12:10.

This book is complementary to my *A Primer of Medicine* (1984, 5th edition, Butterworths) which deals mainly with how to examine patients. This second edition has been completely rewritten and some new material has been added.

It is, as far as I am aware, the only textbook that instructs how to present cases in clinical examinations, and the techniques advised will also be found helpful for presenting cases at medical society meetings.

This book is written not only for medicals in Britain but also those in other countries, especially The Commonwealth and America. The examination procedures and the main problems for the candidates are very much the same throughout the medical world.

MHP
1985

Hampstead
London NW3

Contents

The purpose of examinations

'The examination system should aim at contributing to the education of students.'

Recommendation of the General Medical Council, 1967.

Examinations should be a potent force determining what students should learn. Examinations should be designed to test not only what candidates know but also how they use that knowledge and their ability and facility to recall it, and how well they can examine patients. Some examiners also claim that an additional importance is an assessment of the candidate's personality. But undoubtedly a primary purpose of all examinations is to set educational standards and to assess which candidates have attained those standards.

An anonymous Australian cynic has described medical examinations as 'partially appropriate tests conducted by partially capable examiners on partially equipped candidates.'

Passing examinations indicates, other than in very exceptional cases, a capacity and willingness to work and the possession of at least a modicum of intelligence. For some, examinations are a necessary stimulus to work harder. For a minority, the shadow of forthcoming examinations is the only effective prod to make them study appropriate textbooks and examine many patients with an adequate thoroughness and care. Undoubtedly examinations galvanize some, if not the majority, into a realization of the necessity for systematized and planned learning. The acquisition of a well-stocked mind is an essential part of any education.

Examinations should never be an end in themselves but each has a specific purpose. The essential purpose of the final qualifying examination is for the protection of the public. The purpose of postgraduate examinations is either to select those considered suitable for further training as specialists or consultants (which is the usual practice in the UK), or to choose those considered ready for appointment to a consultant or specialist post in the near future. The examiner's task is a critical assessment to determine whether the candidates can safely be given the responsibility of care of patients, by ensuring that the candidates have sufficient knowledge, practical skill and experience to enable them to practise their art for the benefit of their patients and not to their detriment. The examiners for their part should be competent to examine on the particular subject and they should perform that duty conscientiously. They should pass only those examinees who are both competent and conscientious. Success, especially in postgraduate examinations, should be a very important factor in selection for promotion.

But it is not always idleness or stupidity or too much time spent on extra-curricular activities that causes some students to fail, even repeatedly. Passing examinations may be difficult for even the most intelligent, the most capable and those most willing to attempt to overcome the handicap of poor teaching. Examination failures are an indictment of the teachers because it is they who have failed their students either by neglect of their teaching duties or because of an inability to teach at least reasonably well. Examinations should be regarded by all the staff of teaching hospitals as a test and guide of their teaching efficiency.

From my long and extensive experience of clinical teaching I have no hesitation in maintaining that clinical teaching is often appallingly bad. That a few succeed in overcoming this handicap of inefficient or even bad teaching is no defence. Too many members of teaching hospitals are too prone to emphasize the defects of present-day students or wrongly blame the examination system but never themselves for the present unsatisfactory state of medical undergraduate and postgraduate education.

There are some professors of clinical medicine who are primarily research workers who want to alter the curriculum so as to include more and more of their own pet subject. For example, there are some who believe that accurate measurement of everything possible is the necessary prerequisite of good medical practice. There are others who make the same claims for the most detailed knowledge of biochemistry in all its complexities. Both groups advocate that more time should be spent on these 'basic sciences' and less on clinical medicine proper. A year's lecture course in mathematics has been seriously suggested for all medical undergraduates. One foreign medical school insists on a compulsory whole year spent learning about computers. To me this is as absurd as the compulsory year devoted to Marxian dialectics insisted upon in some of the communist countries. But if attendance at instruction in such subjects is not compulsory only a few would attend them, unless such talent became an essential prerequisite for entrance to medical schools. Otherwise such teaching would be confined to a supposed élite, which is not the true purpose of medical education, certainly at an undergraduate level. And if no examinations are held in such subjects then those who are not of the élite are unlikely to work hard enough to acquire even a modest competence. If examinations in that subject are compulsory will those who fail be victimized by being held back until they pass?

The argument against examinations

It has become fashionable to decry conventional examinations, especially postgraduate ones. This denigration of examinations is often supported by medical teachers, including professors, especially those who themselves experienced difficulty in passing them. They often follow the fashionable permissiveness of modern society and obey the demands for 'democratization', allowing students, however ignorant they may be, to help organize the curriculum and determine how their progress is assessed. Too much tampering with the wind will lead to a lot of spoilt lambs who will become bad doctors.

'Since the day when the first written paper was set, or the first oral examination undertaken, people have been complaining about the iniquity, the clumsiness, inadequacy, and the inappropriateness of examinations. Yet they are still with us because no better means has yet been suggested of making the assessments which are almost universally admitted to be necessary.' (Professor D. Sinclair of Aberdeen in his excellent book *Basic Medical Education* (1972), Oxford University Press.)

Those who oppose examinations often point to the fact that some distinguished people, especially when young, had difficulty in passing examinations. Amongst given examples are Einstein, Ehrlich, Mendel, and John Hunter. Some would explain this apparent anomaly by using the now fashionable phrase, 'late developers'. No individual examination or examination system can ever be perfect but all candidates should scrupulously avoid any criticism of them until they have passed. The candidate's main aim must always be to pass.

However, many educationalists decry examinations because of their supposed bad effects on students. They are none the less an important concern of students themselves, whether they are motivated by the need to pass or a fear of failure, or a varied and sometimes varying mixture of both. Most students appreciate that the only pragmatic indicator of whether they are succeeding in their ambition to become competent doctors, which should always be their main aim, is an examination system. Moreover, many students of their own accord believe that subjects in which there are no examinations cannot be of much importance.

A further criticism is that examinations usually demand an instant recall of facts, but that complaint is totally unjustified because medical education should always be geared to enable and demand that doctors should be able when necessary to make correct decisions quickly, because such a necessity often occurs in clinical practice and depends essentially on an ability to recall rapidly all relevant facts.

Examinations as regards a few individuals may occassionally operate unfairly, but so do all suggested alternatives. Indeed life itself from birth to death is certain to be blighted sometimes with unfair episodes, but being able to cope with them is an essential ingredient of happy living, the truth of which all doctors will have to convince their patients.

Many candidates overemphasize the part played by luck. Napolean said, 'In war luck is on the side of the heavy battalions,' which may be true of war, but in examinations the better prepared the less the need to rely on luck which can never be depended upon. Luck can never be taught or learnt. Very important should be the realization and acceptance of the undoubted fact that it requires intelligence to take good advantage of any luck. One of the best effects of passing an examination is the liberation from a fear of failing it.

The Royal College of Physicians (London), in 1956, issued a report on medical examinations which stated: 'At all stages of medical education examinations now exercise an unhealthy dominance over the students' work and thought'. If this is truly so then the blame must lie entirely with the medical schools and those institutions that organize undergraduate and postgraduate examinations.

The ever-increasing numbers sitting all medical examinations has undoubtedly caused serious difficulties in arranging and conducting examinations, especially clinicals and other orals. But examiners should never allow such difficulties to be made an excuse for diminishing either the conscientiousness or thoroughness with which they undertake their privileged task. Expediency in such circumstances may legitimately be a minor consideration but must never be of paramount importance. Examiners must see to it that, in spite of all difficulties, Kingsley Amis's gibe, 'more, meaning worse,' does not apply to the number of candidates affecting the quality of the examination.

A further complaint by some is that examinations allow no scope for original ideas. But should a final-year student or even one for a higher degree or diploma be expected to have original ideas, for example, concerning the physical signs of mitral stenosis or frontal lobe tumour, or the technique of gastrectomy, or, indeed, concerning any other clinical matter? Only a minute proportion of the population have ever had an original idea in their lives. Those who make this complaint against examinations are often the same people who are enthusiasts for multiple choice questions in which candidates have to answer a 'yes' or a 'no' and any other reply is considered to be wrong. Is this allowing scope for originality?

Unfortunately, medical examinations have become a large and profitable industry for some authors, publishers and those medical institutions that largely depend on them for their finances. This often leads to wasted studies, ill-afforded finances, and sometimes great unhappiness and even bitterness.

Suggested alternatives

Professors of medicine and others responsible for medical education should be wary of listening to that new breed calling themselves 'medical educationalists', who attempt stridently to sell their theories even although they themselves rarely, if ever, attempt to teach. These peculiar people, nicknamed 'the bother boys' by Dr Derek Myers of Brisbane, Australia, have attempted to impose their conceits and delusions on medical education. There is no evidence that any of their suggestions when acted upon have ever produced better doctors. The 'bother boys' are often motivated by their false convictions that they have not only an ability but also the duty to tell others how to regulate and organize their teaching or learning. They seem to value only what they consider can be measured objectively.

Some medical professors have instituted the replacement of conventional examinations, especially 'finals', by continued or continuing assessments. But such tests are euphemisms for examinations, albeit of a different kind. The late Sir George Pickering wrote, 'The laudable object of monitoring students' progress by continuous assessment has degenerated into frequent examinations'. (*Quest for Excellence in Medical Education* (1978), Oxford University Press.)

Moreover, continuing assessment usually finally depends on written reports by members of the staff on each individual student. But a teacher who teaches only large groups, which is common, is not in a position to give such reports honestly. It is claimed that continuing assessment avoids the emotional stress of traditional examinations, especially 'finals'. But it is very doubtful that this aim is achieved because it merely alters the timing and the frequency and character of possible anxieties. Moreover, it ignores the fact that medical practice will certainly be peppered with many emotional crises, minor and major, with which every doctor must learn to cope. Furthermore, such a viewpoint ignores the undoubted fact that but very few ever face any examination with complete equanimity. Continuing assessment merely converts a possible acute anxiety into a chronic one. Every clinical teacher each time he conducts a ward round or clinic in the presence of students should assess each individual's performance and correct any mistakes or poor techniques of examination of patients, and this is a laudable form of continuing assessment.

Students should not be cajoled into using so-called 'self-assessment' methods, whether multiple choice questions or problem solving, and their use, if any, should be left to those who enjoy doing them voluntarily. Certainly, their educational value has never been proved. They are sometimes an excuse for seniors to reduce their teaching to a bare minimum. They often cause time to be wasted in libraries which would be far better spent examining patients. Different schools use different assessment techniques and make different uses of their own results.

A false assumption is often accepted that definite criteria for the satisfactory performance of assessment tests have been established and complied with and that students know those criteria. Continuous assessment smacks of Big Brother and Big Brother may be much more interested in, for example, students' extra-curricular activities, than in medical abilities.

Another fashionable procedure is the setting of 'problem solving' questions in which a very limited and grossly inadequate (although often containing many irrelevancies) medical history is given together with a few selected physical signs and investigations (also often irrelevant) concerning a patient, nearly always a fictitious one. Clinical examinations of all types should always have a very definite and close relationship with actual medical practice, which such tests rarely possess. Good bedside teaching includes discussion on solving diagnostic problems. But when such problems are confined to a printed page responsibility is placed entirely on the student, the teacher no longer playing his traditional role but acting essentially at best as manager and at worst merely as a distributor of leaflets.

If postgraduate medical examinations are abolished, as some advocate, what, if anything will replace them? The greatest danger is that promotion will depend entirely on the senior proclaiming loudly and frequently that his junior, his apprentice, his servile stooge, deserves promotion for no other valid reason than that he has worked for him. Promotion may also depend on how influential and free from personal enemies his chief is. But the chief is rarely an unbiased assessor of his junior's true clinical ability. The junior must rigidly follow his senior's research and specialist interests. It may occur that the senior says of his assistant, as I often heard in the army, 'This man should go far and the sooner he starts going the better,' resulting in false praise. But what if after a long apprenticeship during which the junior has served the senior faithfully and worked hard, even doing many of the tasks that the senior himself should have done but neglected, the chief suddenly takes a dislike to his junior, probably for some trivial non-medical reason. He may become aware that his junior has developed halitosis, or has had some success with a damsel who has rebuffed the senior's advances. Or he, the senior, may belatedly discover that his apprentice formerly was a member of a communist of fascist party. So, despite long diligent service the apprentice loses his chief's support, so vital to his promotion.

The truth is that the medical fate of many junior doctors is in the hands of some consultant who can make or break them, which they often do most unscrupulously. Those who campaign for the abolition of examinations often want a complete mastery over those serving them. Promotion then depends mainly, if not completely, on their juniors being smug, sycophantic and conforming. In some teaching hospitals, athletic prowess counts enormously, and such extraneous factors may be considered more important than clinical ability. But too much agreement with authority and the development of 'yes-men' must inevitably lead to mediocrity and the bland leading the bland. Those who have done well in examinations should have some valid claim to promotion even if they fall foul of their chief.

'One thing is certain, if teachers taught more and conducted examinations less, the students would learn more. If we need to add anything further to the medical curriculum it is spare time'. (Grains and Scruples (1938). *Lancet.*) Medical students need plenty of time for quiet study on their own, including actually dealing with patients, which may mean fewer organized classes and lectures than is common today in many teaching hospitals.

2

Preparation for examinations

'Do not say, when I have leisure I will study, because perhaps you never will have leisure'.

(Talmud. Perke Avot 2).

Study

The first preparation for any examination is to make sure that you are fully and correctly informed about the regulations and the way the examination is conducted. This may mean writing to the appropriate secretary of the examining board and asking about the regulations, and if you yourself are eligible, the dates of the examination, and any other details which may be available.

Nobody, however brilliant, ever got through medical examinations without hard work. Studying is a habit which you must acquire and disciplining yourself is an essential prerequisite to success.

No student can know a subject adequately unless he has studied it sufficiently. Regular periods of well-arranged and concentrated study are the hallmark of the well-ordered mind. Such study cannot possibly be assisted by distractions such as background music, or television, or extraneous conversation. A quiet place of study which is neither too hot nor too cold and free from noise and possible interruptions should be sought.

Each student is a law unto himself or herself as to the best methods of preparation, depending on the individual's personality and different cognitive styles, the various ways in which different people gather and make use of information, using techniques which they have found by experience to suit them personally although their methods may be inimical to others equally intelligent. Undoubtedly an awareness of areas of ignorance should be an essential step towards suitable study.

Extra-curricular activities and interests are essential if you are not to become a stupendous bore, incapable of any serious non-medical conversation, or knowledge of art, music, non-medical literature and foreign travel. But such activities must be indulged in moderately, forming only a comparatively minor part of your life until you have passed the examination, and they must never be an excuse for neglecting studies. This may mean some curtailment of social activities, but that price is well worth paying if it helps towards an early pass rather than protracted preparation or several failures.

It is important that you never attempt an examination for which you are knowingly ill prepared, which would abnegate any possibility of confidence. In such circumstances do not waste your money on entrance fees for the examination, fees that nowadays are often very high. Failure, even when expected, can be very demoralizing. Unfortunately, for various spurious reasons some seniors wrongly encourage their students to sit examinations, especially postgraduate, for which they are ill prepared.

An important aspect of learning is a desire to learn. Do not exhibit a willingness to take everything from your teachers and parents except advice. Knowledge and technical ability are not acquired by inspiration but only by study and the frequent practice of the technical aspects of medicine, especially the seeking out of clinical signs and their correct interpretation. It has become fashionable to decry factual knowledge but this attitude is at best unhelpful and, at worst, stupid. It is impossible to be a good doctor without possessing a large store of factual knowledge.

A frequent recitation of facts, what pedagogues used to call 'learning by rote,' is a method of learning which is despised by many so-called 'educationists'. But it is often an excellent way of remembering the comparatively limited number of 'essential' facts. This is the type of information that cannot possibly be derived from reasoning or deliberation and has no relationship to logic, understanding, or any other ratiocinative process. Those whose auditory memory far exceeds their visual memory may benefit from putting such information on tape and frequently playing it for short periods, especially when reading is inappropriate.

Training in clinical medicine should entail practice under skilled and genuine supervision. This is what is meant by good teaching. A good teacher will not only recognize his students' mistakes as mistakes but will also insist that serious endeavour be made not to repeat them. Wrong ideas and bad techniques should be discovered and corrected at an early stage in a career because if persisted in for long they are very likely to prove difficult or even impossible to correct and eradicate. If for years you have played a skilled game, such as golf or tennis, or a musical instrument, persistently using faulty methods, then it is extremely unlikely that you will ever be good at that game or playing that instrument. Proficiency is likely to be achieved only if early training is good, and that means practice with the guidance of others who supply both instruction and criticism.

In your preparations do not avoid any subject that you do not like, gambling in the hope that in an examination you will be asked little or nothing concerning those subjects that you dislike or find difficult. Far more reasonable to devote extra time and special attention to your dislikes and failings. You should always be conscious of your deficiencies of knowledge and clinical ability and attempt to reduce those gaps and improve those technical abilities, for example, cardiac auscultation or ophthalmoscopy, by frequent practice. Spinoza in his *Ethics* wrote, 'As long as a person declares that he cannot do a certain thing, so long is it impossible for him to do it'.

Reading

'Hear them, read much, learn and inwardly digest'.
Book of Common Prayer, 2nd Sunday in Advent

When reading medical textbooks or journals it is important to differentiate between first what is essential and necessary knowledge, secondly what is inessential but may possibly be useful, and thirdly what is merely ornamental. You must try to attain complete mastery of the information belonging to the first category before attempting to learn much within the second group and before trying to memorize or even understand anything of the third category. Obviously these cannot ever be water-tight compartments 'but most medical information can readily and unequivocally be placed within this scheme. Most important of all considerations must always be that facts gain precedence over theories. The hope is that your teachers have put everything into correct perspective for you and either informed you, or at least given clear indications, as to what should be definitely included in each of the above three categories.

Be not amongst those who leave all meaningful study until a week or two before the examination. This is neither conducive to good results nor to the development of a suitable and sensible attitude towards examinations.

There are two classes of readers, those who read to remember, and those who read to forget. Illiteracy is deplorable but is never so harmful as believing everything read. Especially young undergraduates and young graduates have great difficulty, or even find it impossible, to assess the relative importance and reliability of a great deal of medical literature. 'Not even a dog catcher can learn his trade from books but only from experience. And how much more is this true of the physician'. (Paracelsus, 1493-1541). Do not waste time attempting to master or even understand the gobbledegook contained in most medical journals, or even bother to skim through them. Read only selected material that is most likely to be relevant to the examination which you intend to sit. This nearly always means avoiding what Americans call 'hot medicine,' the latest outpourings studded with statistics and biochemistry which is medical science fiction masquerading as truths. Undoubtedly there is a vast amount of effete and worthless material in recent medical literature, which, like the outpourings of many theologians, consists of the discussion of the undiscussable, and is of no practical value.

Specialist textbooks limited to a single branch of medicine should be avoided unless the postgraduate examination deals entirely with that specialist subject. Bacon in his *Essay on Studies* advised, 'Some books are to be tasted, others to be swallowed, and some few to be cherished and digested'. Certainly every student should be critical when choosing textbooks and the final selection must depend mainly on the nature of the examination and the required standard expected, which will obviously differ, for example, for undergraduate and postgraduate examinations.

It is better to try first to master an elementary smallish book rather than to start with a large tome. But after mastering that small volume a larger textbook should be read to enlarge on the knowledge already acquired and to plug some important gaps which must of necessity have been omitted in the smaller book. How much of the larger volume will have to be carefully studied and learnt will depend on the nature of the examination. For example, as regards clinical medicine I advise Davidson's *Principles and Practice of Medicine* (1984, 14th edition) initially, to be followed by either Cecil's, Harrison's, or Weatherall's much more comprehensive tomes on general medicine. Clinical medicine deals primarily with history taking and the eliciting and interpretation of physical signs but these are neither adequately described nor discussed in modern textbooks of general medicine, and therefore a book dealing mainly and fully with these subjects is essential. I am biased but strongly recommend my own *A Primer of Medicine* (1984, 5th edition, Butterworths).

Many books have recently been published with lists of multiple choice questions and others with collections of alleged problem cases, but in those which I myself have read, the supposed correct answers given are often at best questionable, sometimes misleading, and even occasionally definitely wrong, which is unforgivable. They are nearly always compiled by relatively very inexperienced doctors and are not to be recommended.

Physical fitness

All examinations demand a fair degree of physical fitness. Neither the tired nor the jaded can ever do themselves justice. Immediately before any examination you must have adequate rest and sleep, and, in this context, adequate often means more and not less than usual. Last-minute study, especially if this entails staying up late, is inimical to a good examination performance. If you must turn night into day then you must get adequate food and sleep during the rest of the 24 hours. Why not, if at all possible, spend the weekend prior to an examination away from all study and medical companions intent on nattering about medicine? Juvenal's dictum, 'mens sana in corpore sano' *(Satires* 10, verse 356) may perhaps not be entirely to the liking of modern youth who may be suspicious of some of its implications, but there is undoubtedly much truth in this advice.

It is absurd to have an intensive social life for the greater part of the year and then expect yourself to acquire at least the minimum of requisite knowledge by hectic study a few weeks before the actual examinations. Nobody expects any student to work for 365 days of the year or anything approaching that figure but a sensible plan is to study seriously for, if possible, five nights per week for about 40 weeks of the year and have all other times completely free from medical studies. All students are well advised never to study at weekends unless they have been unable to do so during the week, and never habitually work after about 11 p.m.

Anxiety

Some students, afraid that anxiety may produce, immediately prior to any examination, unpleasant symptoms such as insomnia, gastro-intestinal disturbances, headache, frequency of micturition, etc., may be tempted to take prophylactic tranquillizers or hypnotics. This may turn out to be an ill-conceived practice, especially if you are not used to such self-medication. In spite of the claims of the advertisements, no hypnotic, tranquillizer or sedative has ever been invented that is not liable to produce some hangover, resulting in drowsiness and memory impairment, especially of recall. It is no use ensuring a good sleep the night before an examination if you do not wake up properly until after the examination is half over. Physical rest is in itself, even if accompanied by little actual sleep, preferable to that. On the other hand do not go to bed too early on the eve of an examination in the hope that you will get an extra-long sleep. This may increase anxiety and wakefulness if you do not go to sleep soon after going to bed, because the time may be unprofitably spent worrying about the forthcoming ordeal.

Anticipated symptoms, such as those listed above, which recur before or during each examination are indicative of anxiety which is usually engendered by at least a suspicion that preparation for the test has been insufficient. This may appear to be a harsh judgement, for example, on a migraine sufferer, but it is often a true description of the situation. There are hardly any who go into an examination without some degree of anxiety and this appreciation that everybody else is also anxious should comfort you. Complete absence of anxiety usually indicates a smugness and complacency which is often not justifiable, or that the candidate is not taking the examination as seriously as he should. The remedy should never be reliance on a drug taken at the eleventh hour but an entirely different approach to the examination, including adequate preparation for it.

Examination phobias must be recognized as irrational. Furthermore, you must never allow yourself to be disturbed, with consequent anxiety, by accounts given to you by those who have failed that examination. Their excuses for their failures are nearly always spurious. A person of only moderate ability may actually be a good candidate if he avoids all unnecessary anxiety and thereby displays self-confidence. The best way to acquire and later show such self-confidence is a critical awareness that you have a sound knowledge of the subject.

Nattering about the forthcoming battle often produces anxiety, so immediately before any examination avoid the company of fellow candidates who insist on discussing subjects about which you might be asked. To be informed at such a late hour of things of which you are ignorant is likely to militate against the sang-froid and self-confidence for which you should strive.

Special preparation for oral examinations

Undoubtedly, medical students these days are not subjected to the intensive questioning and quizzing to which they often were in the past. As a result of this many students are unused to being questioned in a critical way, or being contradicted, or being asked to justify and explain everything they have said, or confidently being able to demonstrate with good techniques how they elicited positive and negative physical signs.

Since they are not used to being bombarded with searching questions, such treatment in an examination is too novel and devastating an experience. This inability of many students to stand up to reasonable questioning I regard as another indication of the poorness or failure of present-day medical education.

I strongly advise that you form quiz groups of about four from amongst your colleagues and practise the art of verbal answers. But be careful whom you choose as members of your group and avoid smart alecs who insist in asking absurd or abstruse questions, often in an attempt to demonstrate their own supposed cleverness.

Another excellent preparation for orals is the judicious use of a tape recorder. Get a respected friend or senior colleague to write out suitable questions, each of which can be fairly completely answered within 3-5 minutes. Each question is written out on a different piece of paper which is later folded. At the appropriate time you should then open one of the folded pieces of paper and immediately start talking into the tape recorder and speak for a timed 3-5 minutes. Later, with the playback your deficiencies, such as long periods of silence, waffling and evasions, hesitations, lack of logical sequences of expression, frequent 'ums' and 'ers' and the like, poorness of elocution, and actual lack of knowledge of the subject, may all become apparent. A tape recorder properly used can be an excellent teaching aid and an exposé of faults. Your task will then be to work hard to correct those faults.

Correct attitude and motivation towards examinations

Whatever the reader's personal views are about examinations in general and of any particular examination it is important to adopt a sensible attitude. A correct frame of mind is essential, looking upon passing medical examinations as at worst a necessary nuisance, or as hurdles which must be successfully negotiated. They should always be regarded as a challenge which is to be readily accepted as such without moaning or complaints. A determination to succeed must dominate your thoughts and influence your actions. Singleness of purpose is essential. Correct motivation, including the determination to pass, is of tremendous importance. You must have a strong and irrepressible desire to achieve your objective either to become a qualified doctor in the shortest possible time or obtain the higher degree or diploma necessary for ascent of the slippery promotion ladder. Examinations must never be regarded as a barrier between you and paradise or as a means of gaining riches beyond the dreams of avarice.

Each examination has its own peculiar facets and pitfalls and the candidate should attempt to find out from well-informed sources the precise way that that particular examination is conducted, the relative importance of different topics, and, if possible, the methods of marking and assessment. But be careful and discriminating concerning those from whom you seek such information. Do not be frightened by the exaggerations of those who have failed. Their distorted accounts are their own personal excuses for their failures. The examinee must always strive to follow and obey the rules and conventions of the particular examination. The candidate who keeps on moaning and complaining about the stupidities and unfairness of an examination is rarely successful. You must be prepared to triumph over any stupidities and unfairnesses. A pragmatic attitude, a determination to overcome all possible obstacles, is essential.

Unfortunately, especially in postgraduate examinations, it may be very difficult or even impossible for candidates to obtain wholly reliable and correct information about important details of how the examination is actually conducted and marked. Unfortunately, Establishment institutions often thrive on secrecy and owe much of their power to it, but this results in great difficulty, and even the frequent impossibility, of obtaining accurate information concerning the examinations which they conduct.

Advice obtained from self-styled experts and those who claim to have knowledge of the inner workings of some medical institutions, or acquaintanceship with those very limited few who actually have that knowledge, should be regarded with suspicion, because rarely it is either valuable or authentic and it may even be unintentionally bad. There are too many who try to bolster their supposed importance by claiming to have inside knowledge which in fact they do not possess, and their advice is often impracticable or even misleading.

Especially for some postgraduate examinations you may have to travel a considerable distance from your home. Make sure that you will be in the right place at the right time. If the distance is very large it may be preferable or even necessary to stay nearby overnight. All rail or air times of departure and arrival must be carefully checked as no excuses will ever be accepted for late arrival.

A final point which may help some of you during the period of preparation, especially those from abroad whose concentration on study is disturbed by feelings of home-sickness. A partial corrective may be the frequent use of the telephone or tape-recorder cassettes to send and receive frequent messages to and from your family and friends, the spoken voice often being more acceptable and meaningful than the written word.

3

Examiners

'Examinations are a formidable task even to the best prepared,
for the greatest fool may ask more than the wisest man can
answer.'

Charles Caleb Colton. *Lacon,* Volume I

There are three principal components of an examination: (1) the
candidates; (2) the material, namely, the actual questions asked
and things shown, such as specimens, X-rays, laboratory reports
and patients; and (3) the examiners. A very few candidates are
very good and will pass whatever the nature and quality of the
other two components. A number, which unfortunately is always
larger than the previous group, will definitely fail, however helpful
and considerate the examiners. But the greatest number will be
those who perform indifferently and are consequently borderline.
Most of these are given the benefit of the doubt when the
examiners consider whether to pass them, which is probably a
satisfactory state of affairs for undergraduate examinations.

Most examiners are considerate and try to help candidates
especially to overcome any immediate nervousness, and most are
prepared to overlook omissions or minor errors which they
consider to be definitely due to the candidate's anxiety, but such
allowances cannot be relied on. But there are also indifferent and
bad examiners and this is always a deplorable state of affairs.
Examining is both an art and a special skill which unfortunately
few medicals possess. Examinations sometimes more accurately
measure the abilities of the examiners themselves rather than
those of the candidates. 'Examinations measure examiners' (Sir
Walter A. Raleigh, professor of English, Liverpool in *Laughter
from a Cloud* (1923)). The value and fairness of all examinations
depends mainly on those who set and those who mark them. The
bad examiners should be eliminated either by a more critical
selection or by an insistence that all potential examiners pass an
equivalent examination immediately prior to their being entrusted
with the honour and responsibility. But persons who themselves

fail such tests ought not to become or remain examiners, otherwise the tests become merely a game or even a lark with no possible bad consequences. This is an example of the intellectual dishonesty that is rife in some medical schools.

The super-specialist or the man who has attained eminence because of a gimmick is very likely to be a pedant who idolatrously worships his narrow subject or gimmick, who exaggerates the importance of his technical jargon, who prides himself on his mastery of the trivia and minutiae of his small subject, and who, if he is an examiner, would consider lack of such knowledge a grievous defect. His own zeal, dogmatism and narrow expertise render him an unsatisfactory examiner and should disqualify him from holding such office.

Clinical examinations at all levels, undergraduate and postgraduate, should be arranged and conducted by real clinicians and never by those who are primarily research workers who are only dabbling in clinical medicine. Perhaps better to allow an inanimate one-opinion computer to conduct examinations rather than a pompous, self-opinionated super-specialist. Super-specialists should never be allowed to play any important role in either the final qualifying examination or higher qualifications, except in a few highly specialized ones. It is significant that quite a few examiners for Membership of the Royal College of Physicians themselves repeatedly failed that examination and in some instances never even succeeded in passing the examination but were later elected without examination. Some may praise the perseverance of those doctors but repeated failure must cast doubts on their ability, both as examiners, and examinees. This is another example of intellectual dishonesty at its most brazen.

All examiners should seriously endeavour never to be irascible or difficult. Very few examiners in fact are likely to be bad tempered or unfair. On the other hand, there are some who are inclined to be generous, a few even over-generous with their marks; and some are, on the contrary, stingy and hypercritical. All examiners should be aware of their own foibles, hobby-horses, and even ignorances, and, if necessary, these should be pointed out to them by their colleagues. Many bad examiners fall into one of three ornithological categories. First, the woodpecker who relentlessly hammers away at a small object. Secondly, the cuckoo who relies completely on others to do the necessary preparatory work, for example, accepting summaries of the patient's signs without checking either their source or accuracy. Thirdly, the peacocks whose main concern is to impress their fellow examiners.

Any examiner who frequently complains that being an examiner is boring should be removed from the examining panel. Senility should also be a bar. A surprising historical fact is that Sir William Lawrence at the age of 84 was still examining for the Royal College of Surgeons and still operating at St. Bartholomew's Hospital, London.

It is right for examiners to allow candidates to talk without interruption but they should interfere if the candidate is waffling, or reciting an apparently endless list of negative findings, or talking nonsense, or is completely off the correct diagnostic wavelength. However, some examiners seem to delight in pushing candidates who have said something hopelessly wrong further and further up the garden path and finally sinking them in the mire, instead of giving them a chance of correcting themselves at the outset, or the examiner changing the subject. Other examiners are bad because they terrify candidates by frequent unnecessary interruptions or putting their questions badly. Other examiners talk far too much, giving the candidates very little time to reveal their knowledge. Other examiners like to air their own supposed erudition and supply information which is sometimes completely phoney, especially as regards theories of aetiology or medical etymology or details of medical biographies. In all such circumstances the candidates should listen attentively, even feigning great interest, and thank the examiner for the information supplied.

According to his grandson biographer, the very remarkable Sir Jonathan Hutchinson gave a lecture in 1895 in Liverpool in which he proclaimed that he sympathized with candidates rather than with examiners, and that he himself when examining always tried to eliminate any personal element. He pointed out that the state of health and temper of the examiner and any differences or similarities of temperament between examiner and examined might count for too much. He himself tried to eliminate chance and considered it grossly unfair for any examiner having found a student's weak spot to follow it up to damnation, and equally unfair to continue to ask questions only on his own narrow subject.

4

Candidates' relations with examiners

A spokesman for the Royal College of Physicians, Dr Badenoch, in 1962 maintained that its examinations were: 'intended to measure not how good a doctor a candidate is, but how suitable he is for specialist training. . . . Some people one would not want to be a Member of the Royal College'. Such a viewpoint and acting upon it is likely to lead to great abuse because of irrational prejudices, and his failure to describe the alleged undesirable qualities is ominous. Assessment of clinical ability should be the prime, if not the sole, aim of such examinations.

Especially nowadays, when it has absurdly become fashionable in clinical examinations, including those for higher degrees and diplomas, to show patients with few or even no positive physical signs, or patients with no real diagnostic problem, or those cases which over 90% of the candidates diagnose correctly without any difficulty, then the decision whether to pass or fail any candidate often depends on completely extraneous factors rather than satisfactory replies to relevant questions. So immediately getting on good terms with examiners and remaining in that happy state is more than ever necessary, even obligatory. The very least you can attempt to do is not say or do anything or act in any way that may possibly arouse even the slightest adverse criticism from any of the examiners, not even a single one. Examiners, however provocative they may be, should never be regarded by candidates as enemies, ogres or fools, and neither examiners nor examinees should regard examinations as battle confrontations, the 'us' against 'them' attitude.

Dress

'Costly thy habit as thy purse can buy,
But not expressed in fancy; rich, not gaudy;
For the apparel often proclaims the man.'

Hamlet Act I scene 3.

Some examiners falsely claim to be able to assess candidates after only a few minutes' acquaintance. This nearly always depends on a rapid, illogical and often wholly unfair immediate like or dislike of a candidate. So, you must see to it that at least your personal appearance is unlikely to offend anybody. Your dress must be neat and sober, not trendy, exotic or eccentric. A dark lounge suit with well-pressed trouser, white shirt and sober tie should be worn. Club ties sometimes cause snide remarks so are not advisable. Shoes must be well polished and hands and nails must be meticulously clean. It is now fashionable to have long hair but, however much it may offend your ego, however much you may resent interference with your personal freedom of choice, you must pocket your pride and get your hair cut a few days before the examination. Moreover, the knowledge that you are dressed properly for the occasion may improve your self-confidence. Some examiners will regard it as a personal insult if your dress and appearance do not befit the occasion.

Female candidates may have some difficulty in choosing their attire, perhaps finding it difficult to achieve a judicious balance between sex appeal and 'professional sobriety'. Cosmetics and perfumes must be used sparingly and nail varnish is usually frowned upon. They should not wear heavy bracelets, or dangling ear rings or necklaces.

It is imperative that you have a correct attitude towards the examiners, the great majority of whom are out to help candidates and not to fail them. Never regard examiners as enemies, because to do so is likely to produce a bad examiner–examinee relationship. The majority of examiners are pleasant, fair and helpful and are not sarcastic or sadistic, and they try to put candidates at their ease. Neither should you regard all questions as tricks, as such an attitude is likely to lead you to give absurd replies to even the most elementary of questions. You must assume, at least initially, that all examiners are experts on the subject about which they are questioning you.

Bad habits

Ask yourself if you have any bad habits which any examiner may find in any way objectionable. Perhaps it may be more profitable to ask your colleagues especially your seniors, whether they have any criticism of your habits when talking. These are habits of which many are themselves unaware, such as snorting and hawking or making other objectionable noises; nail biting;

scratching some part of the anatomy; keeping fingers or even the whole hand over the mouth when talking; and putting hand or hands in pockets. You are likely to come into fairly close proximity with the examiners during oral examinations so be careful that immediately prior to the event you do not partake of alcohol or strongly smelling foods such as garlic, onions or curries. Do not let your joy of tasty foods leave a pungent odour to your breath.

Never argue with or contradict any examiner, or ever give even the slightest impression of doing so. Never attempt to justify your mistakes but be prepared to admit that your were wrong, even that you have talked nonsense, and admit it without a hint of an excuse. If you consider the examiner has said something that is undoubtedly false you must not by word or manner betray your true feelings and in such circumstances you must not give your own contrary opinion or quote anybody, however eminent, in your support. Occasionally an examiner is pleased and gives special credit to a candidate who teaches him something, but then this must always be attempted in a diplomatic and circumspect fashion, devoid of the slightest trace of aggression, condescension or patronization. Generally speaking, it is not the candidate's duty to educate any examiner or the examiner's duty to teach the candidates. For several years I personally have spent much time and energy denouncing 'bull' in our profession but all candidates must be pragmatic and realize that for many of them a modicum of bluff and blarney may be essential for their success.

Self-confidence

'He heals best in whom most people have the greatest confidence.'

Galen – Greek physician, CE 130–200, who emigrated to Rome in CE 160.

Galen's aphorism applies equally to the relationship between candidates and examiners. You must attempt to ooze self-confidence and avoid at all costs even the slightest hint of its lack. The following advice is given to help you convey such an attitude.

Your facial expressions are often the main indication of your self-confidence or lack of it. An occasional smile is always a great help. On the other hand, do not go to the other extreme and display a continuous smirk or grin which an examiner may misinterpret or find irritating. Many candidates betray an air of constant apprehension, acute misery, or even terror. You must be determined not to exhibit any stigmata of gross anxiety or fright. Tears never win marks, even if shed by the most attractive woman, but are likely to produce acute embarrassment in the examiner with consequent resentment. Do not over-compensate any feelings of worry or anxiety by an apparent aggressiveness in manner or speech.

5

Essay questions

The opposition to essay questions

Following continued pressure over a number of years many of those who are responsible for organizing and conducting medical examinations have yielded to the propaganda against the essay type of written questions, and have either abolished written papers altogether or replaced them by multiple choice questions (MCQ). Typical of this anti-essay lobby is Dr Bull, formerly Professor of Medicine at Belfast.

Professor Bull whose main interest, judging by his research publications, appears to be mathematics rather than clinical medicine, wrote in *The Lancet*: 'There is a considerable element of error in marking long essay questions, but the error diminishes progressively as the questions (sic) are shortened'. He meant 'answers' and not 'questions', but an interest in mathematical accuracy does not often coincide with an interest in literary accuracy.

A logical inference from his statement could be that when written answers are reduced to a monosyllable or even a single sign as they are in MCQ tests then the perfect questions have been set. Moreover, his statement does not require any statistical survey such as he supplied to support the thesis that very long essays are very difficult to assess unless the examiner has at his disposal unlimited time for reading and marking them. A more valid and useful inference from his own statistics is that the wrong questions are often set.

The late Sir George Pickering, formerly Professor of Medicine at St. Mary's London and later at Oxford, spent a good deal of his time touring the world talking about medical education without himself achieving any renown as a medical teacher. He wrote in *The British Medical Journal* of July 1956:

> 'Written papers seem designed not to test a student's capacity to discriminate but his capacity to reproduce material learned from the pages of a textbook or the notes of lectures. The kind

of question which is still current in the final examination in medicine is a question such as, "Describe the symptoms, signs and complications and the treatment of ulcerative colitis" .'

Whose fault is it that such questions as that cited by the Professor are ever asked? There is something perverse about those who denounce such questions as if it were not they themselves and their colleagues who are responsible for setting such questions. To me the fault with such a question is that it demands too much information so that most candidates will write reams and reams and then Professor Bull and his followers will be able to prove from some further statistical survey that the various examiners marking that question will give a wide range of marks. It is the examiners who set such questions who are at fault, for not having either the knowledge or the time to devise better questions demanding more limited and more concise answers. On the other hand I would not support those who in a qualifying examination would replace the question quoted by Sir George by, for example, 'Discuss the theories of aetiology of ulcerative colitis' or the even more esoteric question, 'Discuss the role of immune mechanisms in the aetiology of ulcerative colitis'. May students be spared such examiners.

In a subject such as clinical medicine written questions should never be of a kind that can be satisfactorily answered from consecutive pages of some standard textbook, but should be those that require the application and redaction of information which is scattered over many pages of several appropriate textbooks. To give but two suggested questions which I regard as suitable for a qualifying examination:

1. A middle-aged patient complains of progressive difficulty in walking and on examination is found to have absent ankle jerks and extensor plantar responses. Discuss the differential diagnosis.
2. A patient complains of recent severe headache and epistaxis and has a temperature of 102 and purpura. Discuss the differential diagnosis.

The truth is that many examiners are not prepared to think out and formulate such questions. It is sheer laziness and perverseness on their part to set such a question as that cited by Sir George and then complain that the answers are so long that they cannot be assessed accurately. The setting of examination questions is a serious and very important aspect of education. It is too often forgotten that it is the organizers of examinations who decide what is worth while in education. By the quality of their examination questions teachers should be known and judged. Questions should test not only the range and depth of knowledge but also the ability to organize and express facts and ideas lucidly, and this can be achieved in written papers only by the essay type of questions. I do not entirely approve of the common practice nowadays of marking within a very narrow range such as 45–60% and claiming a scientific basis for this, because of its reputed lowering of the correlation between the marks awarded and the candidate's real ability.

Advice on answering essay questions

Always first make sure that you have carefully complied with all the requirements regarding name and/or examination number, and any other information asked for. Afro-Asians should be careful that they give their names exactly and in the identical order as they did on their application forms to sit the examination.

Much of the advice on how to answer written questions applies equally forcibly to oral answers. Success does not depend entirely on memory but rather on the presentation of such knowledge as you possess (which may be minimal but yet sufficient) in good order, and making the best display of that knowledge.

Unless informed otherwise you must always assume that each question will carry the same number of marks. So divide the total time allotted for the whole paper by the number of questions to be answered. If there are four questions to be answered in 3 hours, then about 45 minutes must be spent on each question, and never more than a few minutes over that time. It is foolish to spend more than this on any individual question and skimp others. Even if you wrote a 'perfect' answer to any individual question the probability is, especially the way questions are marked nowadays, that your score will be less than 70% for that 'perfect' answer. But this will be of no avail if you get a very low mark on one or more of the other questions. Any question that you consider to be difficult should demand at least the full time because you will have to think more, as the relevant points will not come so readily and you will be hesitant. In some examinations it is expected, perhaps even demanded, that a pass mark be obtained for each individual written question.

If you have to answer all the questions, that is, if no selection is allowed, I strongly advocate the following technique. Before even glancing at any of the questions cover up all of them except the first and answer that for the calculated time, without previously looking at any of the other questions. When that time is up, immediately finish with that answer and uncover the second question. Follow this method with each question in turn. The reason why I so strongly advise this method is for the necessity to concentrate on each individual question one at a time. If you start by reading through the whole paper as is often recommended this will almost certainly result in you attempting to think about several questions at once, with resultant disturbance of your concentration on the question you are answering. Worrying about any question other than the one you are answering will militate against the cool calm concentration so vital in all examinations, including written ones.

Moreover, when all questions are compulsory it is stupid to waste time trying to decide on the order in which you will write the answers. So, as advised, when no choice is allowed, answer the questions in the order they appear on the paper. By this method you are also more likely to distribute the time equally for each question. If, however, you are allowed a choice then of course you must read through them all, but this should be done quickly and a rapid decision made on your selection. Time must never be wasted on selection. Furthermore, once you have started to write an answer, only in very exceptional circumstances should you ever change your mind and abandon that question in favour of another.

When allowed a choice always pick the question about which you can write most rather than one about which you may know a great deal in terms of the percentage of recorded facts but about which the total amount you can write is very limited. For example, always prefer a question such as, 'Describe the manifestations of sarcoidosis', even though you may be well aware of the fact that your answer will be far from complete, rather than a question such as, 'Describe the manifestations of pseudo-xanthoma elasticum' about which you may even be a genuine expert. Always prefer a general question rather than one on a small single facet of a subject. For example, choose 'Discuss the manifestations of uraemia' rather than a question on some narrow specific aspect of renal disease, such as the biochemical consequences of tubular defects.

When selecting questions avoid whenever possible any about which you are not certain exactly what is meant, either because of ambiguity of words or uncertainty as to the meaning of some term. If you appreciate that the meaning of or use of a term used in the question is controversial this in itself is not a valid reason for rejecting that question, provided that you are capable of explaining, for example, the different ways that term is used by different authorities. In fact your information may educate the examiner who should give special credit for such a feat.

Writing a lot

My advice on writing essay answers may be summarized – write a lot! If you cannot succeed by quality you might possibly succeed by quantity. This may sound very cynical but its pragmatism cannot truthfully be gainsaid. Any examiner who informs you that he reads every word carefully, even some claim twice over, is not credible unless he is an unimaginative, under-employed obsessional. I honestly believe that many examiners mark essay questions principally by weight. If you have written a lot then many examiners are likely to come to the conclusion that amongst all that effort there must be much that is good and so are likely to credit the candidate with at least a pass mark. But your writing must always be in lucid, concise and readable prose avoiding jargon, clichés, vague words and phrases, verbosity and prolixity; and its syntax must never either be complex or intrinsically convoluted, or telegraphic, or cryptic, or recorded in abbreviations.

How is this desirable ambition to write a lot to be achieved? First, by *not wasting time* on selection or order of answers, as described above; and secondly by following the advice given under the subheadings below.

No planning

Unfortunately, some people are obsessional planners and not to do so may produce an acute anxiety state. If you belong to this unfortunate tribe then the compulsion to plan must be followed. Planning answers is a grossly overrated and usually ill-advised exercise. Remember that you are not preparing a paper for publication in a learned journal. However knowledgable you are you will never even approximate to a 'perfect' answer because of the contingencies of the examination, including the time limitation.

Furthermore, you either have a plan for a discussion of any particular problem or you do not, and in the latter contingency you are extremely unlikely to think out a satisfactory one during an examination. Any time spent on planning is very likely to be time wasted. If, on the other hand, you know a satisfactory plan there is no point in writing this out on sheets of spare paper. Even more absurd is to work out a plan in rough and then change that plan, especially if you have actually started writing the answer. Such ditherings get you no marks and go against my advice to write a lot. For example, consider the question, 'Discuss the causes of severe persistent headache'. My contention is that it is futile to try to work out or invent a classification if you cannot readily recall one, and it is even more absurd if you have never known one. If you have no plan then start writing immediately with an opening phrase such as, 'An important cause of severe persistent headache is raised intracranial tension' and then expand on the special features of headache in this condition, and the likely associated findings, and then follow this with a discussion of the common causes of raised intracranial tension and the special features of each. Whilst engaged in this exposition it should not be difficult to think of a second cause of severe headache, expressed concisely, which can then be discussed at length in the same way; and then to proceed with third and fourth, etc., causes, always mentioning common causes before rarities.

Sucking a subject dry

This is another important adjunct in your attempt to do yourself justice. You must attempt to write all you know relevant to the subject discussed. You must always suck dry every aspect of each individual topic before you leave it and start on something else. For example, when writing about the manifestations of pyloric stenosis give a full, detailed and as far as possible complete account of each heading such as vomiting, describing all its likely features, before describing another manifestation such as tetany.

Moreover each subdivision of a subject demands a new paragraph.

Some important don'ts

Many examiners mark written questions with the help of a list of points which they consider the candidate should have mentioned. They seek out errors of omission. Too many candidates foolishly consider it their duty and even a virtue to help the examiner to discover readily those errors of omission. But this is not incumbent upon you and it is not in your interest to be so charitably inclined towards examiners. Unless an examiner is blatantly lazy or dishonest he should assume that all the points for which he is seeking in the answer have in fact been included, unless he has definite evidence to the contrary which can be obtained only by reading every word of the answer. You must write your answers with these presumptions in mind. Stated otherwise, your battle cry against the examiners must be, 'It is your job to find out what I have omitted and I am not going to help you in that task because it would be against by own interests'. So, in my list of 'Do Nots' I include the following.

No preliminary tabulations

Under the heading of tabulations I include lists of proposed contents of your answer. I strongly advise against starting an answer to a question about subject X with an opening paragraph such as, 'There are six important factors concerning X' and then naming them. Any examiner who knows several more important factors which he thinks you should have mentioned and discussed may come to the rapid but perhaps unjustified conclusion that you have left several important points out completely, although you may have later included them in your answer.

No headings or underlinings

Headings and underlinings make it too easy for examiners to spot errors of omission. This may be very unfair if inadvertently you have failed to underline some important piece of information or not announced its discussion by a separate heading. Headings and underlinings may indeed help the examiner to assess your answer quickly and more readily but they undoubtedly draw his attention to what you have definitely or probably left out. Your kindness to the examiner may well be at your own expense.

No note-form answers

Most examiners, surprisingly even those who are MCQ enthusiasts, dislike answers written in note form, regarding the practice as the hallmark of the illiterate. Unfortunately, too many medical students and postgraduates are at best semi-literate, but such a serious disability should not be advertised even in an examination.

Another fundamental objection to this type of answer is that the examiner may consider that you have listed things in what you consider to be a correct order of importance. For example, if you have been asked to describe the causes and investigation of recurrent haemoptysis, you may have listed them as follows: 1. Cancer of bronchus; 2. Bronchiectasis; 3. Pulmonary embolism; 4. Pulmonary angioma; 5. Adenoma bronchus, etc. (possibly with an additional 5–10 causes) before realizing that in your compendium you have left out pulmonary tuberculosis. If your answer has been in note form it will be difficult to find a satisfactory solution to your dilemma. Do you completely or partially rewrite the answer? Do you renumber the items with the inevitable untidiness that must result? Do you make substantial alterations which are bound to add to the examiner's difficulty in reading your answer, with consequent annoyance? Whatever your solution it must entail much time wasted. But if you had written your answer in essay form without tabulation, headings or a prologue announcing the subjects you intend to discuss, and you suddenly realized that you had omitted one or more important aspects, you could then start a new paragraph with an opening sentence such as, 'More important than some of the causes mentioned', and then proceed to discuss at length the item or items previously inadvertently left out.

No re-reading

The frequently given advice always to leave time to re-read your answers should never be followed. You are very unlikely to spot any mistakes you have made, including spelling errors. If you have spelt syphilis with an 'f' or pruritus with two 'i's you are very unlikely on any re-reading to spot mistakes. Moreover, it will probably take you over half an hour to read through a 3-hour paper and that time could be far better spent in writing more, especially on those questions which you considered to be exceptionally difficult.

Napolean, Hans Anderson, Sir Joshua Reynolds, George Stephenson, Henry Ford, George Bernard Shaw and Picasso and many others who became famous reportedly had great difficulty in spelling correctly. If you personally are a persistent misspeller the hope is that the examiner will appreciate that this does not invalidate you becoming a competent physician.

No abbreviations

Many examiners object strongly to the use of abbreviations such as MSU, LP, GTT, etc., for certain investigations, and Tb, Sy, LE, MS, AR, AF, CCF, JVP for certain diseases and signs. Avoid all abbreviations whenever possible.

Defining terms and precision of language

> 'How necessary it is for any man who aspires to true knowledge
> to examine the definitions of former authors, and either to
> correct them when they are negligently set out, or to remake
> them for himself.'
>
> Thomas Hobbes (1588–1679), from the chapter Reason and
> Science, in *Leviathan.*

The importance of knowing correct definitions of all the technical
terms used is very important not only in written examinations but
also in orals including clinicals. Indeed, in any oral examination
much time is likely to be devoted asking candidates to explain and
define all terms they may use. It is foolish to use technical words or
phrases, especially new-fangled neolgisms, which you cannot
confidently, quickly and correctly define. Moreover, candidates
must be aware that some terms they may use are controversial and
should be able to discuss why they are controversial, for example,
the term may mean different things to different physicians.
Certainly those who enter any examination neglecting to have
memorized definitions of all the terms which they or the examiner
are likely to use, do so at their peril. Definitions in examinations
are always valuable weapons and reciting them spontaneously is
very likely to impress examiners. But definitions must always be
precise and avoid the use of other words or phrases which
themselves require definition or explanation. In the first published
English dictionary by Samuel Johnson (1709–1784) a cough is
defined as 'a convulsion of the lungs, vellicated by some sharp
serosity' which is an example not to be followed, as is likewise the
clergyman's definition given in a sermon to his congregation, 'An
omer is a tenth part of an ephah'.

Whenever a technical word such as 'nystagmus' or phrase such
as 'extrinsic asthma' is used it should be defined immediately. This
advice also applies to mentions of syndromes. A useful phrase with
which to start such a description is '. . . a condition characterized
by . . . '. Moreover, if such definitions are always automatically
given after mentioning any technical word or phrase orally or in
writing then the good habit may be instilled into you of always
mentioning facts first and leaving out theories until later. For
example, having mentioned Hand–Schüller–Christian syndrome,
immediately state that this is a condition characterized by
deposition of cholesterol material in the skull, together with
exophthalmos and diabetes insipidus, and leave out, at least

initially, any discussion of theories of cholesterol metabolism. This is also an essential method in any oral examination.

Obviously, having defined any term there is no need to repeat it every time that term is used. But you must assume that each question will be marked by a different examiner, so do not hesitate to repeat any definitions given in any previous answer, or to a different examiner in an oral, including clinical.

Illegibility

Illegibility undoubtedly irritates examiners and should whenever possible be avoided. Unfortunately, many medical students and postgraduates cannot write legibly and this disability is extremely difficult if not impossible to correct when writing in examinations. So, any time spent attempting to improve handwriting is not likely to be rewarding unless very many laborious hours are devoted to the task. A suggestion that you submit pages of your writing to a colleague asking him to point out any particular letters or words which he finds especially difficult to interpret, and then concentrate on improving a limited number of your defects, may help. Examiners who set questions demanding lengthy replies are themselves undoubtedly promoting illegibility.

One senior English physician has claimed that he would seriously consider failing any candidate who used a ball-point or similar pen instead of a fountain-pen. Personally I think the use of a good ball-point improves the legibility of some people's writing and is certainly preferable to an unsatisfactory fountain-pen with a nib slightly damaged such as is often used. Moreover, ball-points have the advantage that they rarely leak and do not cause blots, the writing dries quicker and is not easily smudged so that blotting paper is not required, and there is no necessity to carry around a bottle of ink or be worried lest the fountain-pen runs dry. But these are my personal views and it is impossible to give a definite 'yes' or 'no' to the use of ball-points.

Diagrams

The inclusion of diagrams in an answer is excellent provided that they are relevant and can be drawn quickly and reasonably accurately. In qualifying examinations and postgraduate ones this applies especially to neurology; for example, to illustrate the site of a lesion and to name the local anatomical structures involved.

All diagrams must genuinely enlarge upon or make plainer your written description; for example, a line diagram of a cardiac X-ray outline, or reproducing an ECG pattern. You should not attempt to follow many modern textbooks which have line diagrams or even photographs of such procedures as obtaining tendon reflexes or doing a rectal examination. Also, remember that any diagram can too readily show your mistakes, which should not be blatantly exhibited.

Interpretation of some words and phrases commonly used in questions

Often questions begin with one of the following words: discuss, explain, compare, or contrast; and it must be recognized that each of these has a different nuance which must be appreciated.

The word 'discuss' demands an essay type of answer. In other words, it should always be interpreted as meaning, 'Write all you know about'.

The word 'manifestations' when used correctly in clinical medicine should refer solely to symptoms and signs elicited at the bedside. However, in any examination it is prudent to include a brief summary of desirable investigations, but their description must be brief because otherwise they are likely to be regarded as irrelevant.

How to discuss treatment of any condition

If asked to describe the treatment of any condition which has several causes, for example, hypertension, you should first start with a brief mention of at least the common causes and, after each, give a summary of the investigations necessary to prove or disprove each cause. You should then proceed to describe the treatment of the idiopathic condition, be it a syndrome such as Menière's, a symptom such as vertigo, or a clinical entity such as an acoustic neuroma. It is unfortunately true that a few examiners might deem any initial mentioning of known causes as irrelevant, although most examiners are likely to consider such inclusions not only desirable but might penalize you if they were omitted.

When asked to discuss treatment or management of a given condition, a full description of all aspects of therapy is required including, whenever relevant, such matters as diet, rest, advice about occupation, hobbies and recreation, and psychological factors, and, in some instances, indications for surgery.

When mentioning any drug therapy, precise dosage and method of administration must be given and also side effects, toxic reactions and contraindications.

When describing treatment, remember that often surgery must be discussed and the following techniques should be used. Always start with the definite non-controversial indications, then follow with the possibly controversial indications and leave the definitely controversial till the last. For example, when discussing the indications for surgery of a gastric ulcer, first mention perforation, then pyloric stenosis and then strong evidence of malignancy in the absence of definite metastases, and follow that recital with probable, and later possible, indications. In a written paper you should describe, in turn, the basis on which each of these three complications is diagnosed. In an oral examination, after mention of each complication you must be prepared for an intervening question from the examiner asking you for diagnostic details of those complications. After describing these non-controversial indications for surgery of a gastric ulcer you should then mention recurrent haematemesis in a person aged over about 40, which is not an absolute indication but one which should always be seriously considered. Any other indications, such as repeated failure of medical therapy, are left to the last.

Investigations

Strictly speaking the term 'investigation' in clinical medicine should refer to radiological and laboratory procedures. But in any written or oral examination if asked, 'What investigations would you do in a patient with . . . ?' it would be safer to start with a very brief summary of any relevant points in history and clinical signs. For example, in answer to the question, 'How would you investigate a patient with hypertension?', you should start with mentioning enquiry into a family history of high blood pressure, strokes and coronary thrombosis, and a personal history of angina, coronary thrombosis and renal disease. As regards signs in hypertension, mention not only recording blood pressure under various conditions and at various times, but also examination of the fundus oculi and the heart for secondary changes. Then proceed to describe at length the appropriate laboratory and radiological investigations.

When listing suggested investigations obey the following rules. Never merely give a list but after the mention of each individual investigation give the reason for its performance and what you expect it would definitely or probably show. Always start with the simplest investigations and proceed only later to the more and more complex. By simple, I mean not only those easy to perform but also those not presenting any hazards and only minimal discomforts for the patient. For example, when describing investigations of a patient with renal disease start with examination of the urine for protein, casts, red cells, pus cells and organisms and leave such procedures as renal biopsy, renal angiography and ultrasound or computerized axial tomography until later.

Discussion of aetiology

You may be asked to discuss the aetiology of a condition of which the cause is doubtful or unknown. You should discuss all factors that definitely, probably and possibly may have a bearing on the aetiology. Factors to be considered are sex, age, race, occupation and geography. You must also consider any metabolic abnormalities which may have been described in that particular condition and which may possibly be a cause rather than an effect of the disease process. Any organisms which may at any time have been incriminated and possible allergic and immunological factors should be considered. In many conditions, especially those nearly always first manifesting themselves in the older age groups, such as atherosclerosis or osteoarthritis, the aetiology is generally regarded as degenerative due to ageing, which may be premature. The pompous neologism 'cryptogenic' which is now fashionable has no advantage over the long-established word 'idiopathic'.

Use of personal pronoun

Many questions contain the word 'you' but this should not be taken too literally. It is wiser not to use the words 'I', 'we' or 'my' in any answer.

Moreover it may be dangerous to give an account, true or fictitious, of any clinical experience personally observed as this may be considered by the marker to be trite, boastful or untrue. So, unless your experience of a condition is really exceptional and you can explain how that unusual experience came about, it is far better to avoid clinical reminiscences.

6
Multiple choice questions (MCQ)

The USA Board of Internal Medicine adopted MCQ as far back as 1946, but we should not accept this comparatively new system as better than traditional ones merely because it has become fashionable. MCQ have been introduced without any certainty that they are either fair or valid. Many who advocate or actually use them claim that they are a modern, objective, reliable and scientifically valid method of assessment, but they are merely slavishly and uncritically following a fashion. Unfortunately, expediency and not genuine rational evidence has often been the real reason for their acceptance and wholesale introduction.

I personally am strongly opposed to MCQ for medical examinations. They accentuate the unfortunate and undesirable cleavage between the worlds of science and art and make doctors even more than ever incapable of expressing their thoughts accurately and precisely in written and spoken speech when attempting to communicate either with their colleagues or with lay people, especially their patients. One of the most valuable functions of a medical examination should be the assessment of the student's correct use of words, technical and otherwise, and an ability to assemble knowledge in a coherent form. The art of communication and self-expression are of great importance in clinical practice but are ignored by MCQ. Particularly when marked with a computer, MCQ tests feign a scientific accuracy of assessment which they do not intrinsically possess.

All the MCQ tests that I have analysed have been replete with vague words and phrases and ambiguities which are a menace to candidates and a complete abnegation of the claim that they are a scientific mode of assessment. What is meant by words and phrases used in these tests such as, 'common', 'seldom', 'sometimes', 'often', 'rarely occurs', 'known to occur', 'usually occurs', 'seldom occurs', 'typically occurs'? These words and phrases lack both precision and clarity. Is there any difference between 'frequently' and 'very frequently', and other adverbs of number which are often used in these tests? Let me illustrate this by an example taken from an MCQ paper. 'The following conditions are commonly associated with leg ulcers: rheumatoid arthritis; ulcerative colitis; Crohn's disease; polycythaemia vera; sickle-cell anaemia.' Leg ulcers do occur in cases of ulcerative colitis and also of rheumatoid arthritis but does 5%, or thereabouts, constitute 'rarely', 'commonly' or 'frequently' and is such ulceration a complication or an association (a quibble which some delight in)? Having talked to some of the setters of these papers I am sure that to them a 5% incidence or even less should be regarded as 'frequent' or 'common'.

Furthermore, does 'always' really mean in these questions, 'without possible exception'? The same doubt applies to the use of the word 'never'. For example, answering the question, 'Pruritus never occurs in the following: psoriasis; secondary syphilis, etc.', a knowledgeable candidate knowing that pruritus occurs in a small percentage of cases may be tempted to answer 'No', but this will probably be deemed incorrect.

A candidate whom I know to have a fairly wide and sound knowledge of clinical medicine failed the Part 1 MRCP (MCQ examination) probably because he was too accurate, and in answers to questions such as, 'Are the sacroiliac joints *usually* involved in ankylosing spondylitis?', replied 'No'. He claimed that he would have given an affirmative answer only if the question had been worded, 'Are the sacroiliac joints *always* involved in ankylosing spondylitis?

An example from a postgraduate diploma examination was, 'Growth is usually retarded in coeliac disease'. But a correct answer must depend on a knowledge of whether the diagnosis was made early and also if good treatment were given. An example, which curiously is given in the Royal College of Physicians' guide to their own MCQ, is, 'Chronic subdural haematoma frequently presents as fluctuations of consciousness levels and neurological signs'. Is the advised answer 'No' correct? Surely it must depend on some arbitrary meaning of 'frequently'?

MCQ are sometimes themselves long winded containing irrelevant material. At other times the MCQ give such direct clues to the expected answer as to make the test absurdly easy. They sometimes contain abbreviations, acronyms, and eponyms, including controversial examples of each. Sometimes an individual question really consists of two different ones but only one 'yes' or 'no' is required.

MCQ examinations cannot test clinical competence or clinical judgement or conscientiousness, which are all essential qualities for a competent physician. Indeed the more one knows about a subject the more difficult it is often to answer with an unqualified 'yes' or 'no'. Moreover, diagnostic problems do not present in the form suggested by many of these MCQ tests. No patient asks his doctor to tick off from a chosen list the conditions which are the probable cause of his symptoms. MCQ examinations are a deceitful, anti-intellectual and anti-literary 'solution' of the problems that some essay questions create. Setting MCQ is often a shirking of the examiners' responsibilities and this dereliction is accentuated when they do not themselves bother to compose the questions but rely on a 'central bank' to supply them.

In spite of loud cries to the contrary and the supposed safeguards in the system, MCQ engender a guessing competition attitude to medicine and can often be more accurately labelled MGQ (Multiple Guessing Questions). Many MCQ papers have a warning which unjustifiably boasts, 'Guessing will be found out and the candidate penalized'. The subtraction of marks for wrong answers is reputed to prevent guessing being worth while. But such a warning is often a prop to defend a poor method of examination. The whole project is so artificial that every candidate must indulge in at least a modicum of guessing if he is to be successful. For example, asked which organism causes dengue, many would admit ignorance, but if posed in the MCQ format, 'Is dengue due to Group B Arbo-virus?' some would answer 'Yes' because they were really certain that this is true; others reply 'Yes', although they are not certain; others might reply 'No', because although they are certain that an Arbo-virus is the causative organism they mistakenly believe that it is type A; others with a similar doubt may decide to leave the question unanswered because they are uncertain and get no marks; but others may leave the question unanswered because they are completely ignorant on this matter. Another example taken from a postgraduate examination is, 'Filariasis *Wuchereria bancrofti* may cause (a) Calabar swelling (b) lymphangitis (c) a positive serological test for syphilis (d) epididymitis (e) chyluria. The question ignores the fact that the candidate may or may not know that both filariasis and Calabar swelling may be caused by other organisms than the one mentioned. All possible reasons for giving a 'yes' or 'no' answer to many MCQ exhibit different degrees of knowledge or ignorance which cannot be measured by their means. The unfairness of marking such questions demanding a simple 'yes' or 'no' answer when so differing degrees of knowledge may have motivated the answer, illustrates without doubt the farce of the MCQ system.

It has been often stated by MCQ enthusiasts that setting essay questions is easy but marking them fairly is difficult, whilst with

MCQ the reverse is true. But some examiners and medical institutions have found it just as difficult to set MCQ as essay questions and consequently have gladly availed themselves of banks which supply lists of MCQ. The truth is that to set genuinely satisfactory tests of any type requires a great deal of thought and time, which unfortunately many examiners are unwilling to give. MCQ are rarely the objective tests they are claimed to be because their compiling and interpretation are often very subjective and their prior submission to a committee does not necessarily confer objectivity.

Preparation for MCQ tests

My personal views about MCQ tests will not help you to pass these examinations but I hope will reverse their acceptance by examiners. I myself, and several examiners to whom I have spoken, regard these tests as a kind of game akin to crossword puzzles and not to be taken too seriously. But unfortunately candidates must take these seriously if they are to pass.

I know of no certainly useful preparation for these tests other than reading suitable textbooks, preferably large ones, but this does not include those books devoted entirely to MCQ. This is in itself a serious indictment of MCQ because they induce students to spend too much time reading and not enough in the wards examining patients. There can be but little wonder that so many young doctors are very poor clinicians.

So-called model questions issued by correspondence courses, and also published in some medical journals, and in book form, are of very little value because they represent the notions, often very idiosyncratic, of the setter as to what constitutes suitable questions, but his views are very often quite unlike those of the examiners. This arises partly because copies of previously set questions in that particular examination are not available, or only in a very limited form, so the setters of model questions are not aware of the biases and foibles of the examiners. For example, if the setter of such questions had never seen all of the MRCP multiple choice questions set over the past 10 or more years, which is very likely, then he would not credit that von Willebrand disease, gynaecomastia and Conn's syndrome have been great favourites and biochemistry has always played a large part.

Advice on answering MCQ papers

In some MCQ tests the candidates are required to tick those questions to which they consider the correct answer is 'yes' and to leave the others blank. But this is an absurd procedure because an unticked question may either indicate 'no' or 'I do not know' but is marked as though a definite 'no' was meant. It was only after several years of MCQ tests that the Royal College of Physicians realized this obvious fallacy.

Do not go through the whole paper answering only those questions of which you think you are certain of the answer, and then, after re-reading, deciding whether to answer other questions previously left, and perhaps repeating this process several times. Thinking about an answer is unlikely to produce the correct reply in MCQ examinations. For example, if asked, 'Hyponatraemia is a feature of the following: dystrophica myotonica, etc.' no amount of contemplation and cogitation will help and much hesitation is likely to produce dithering with increased anxiety and indecision. Furthermore, first thoughts are often correct and second thoughts often wrong.

Some candidates fail these tests because they mark only those questions about which they are certain. But the fallacy of this is that the candidate is never informed and does not know how many marks he needs to pass. Suppose that there are 60 stem questions each with five branches, constituting in reality 300 questions, and you correctly answer 150, this may be insufficient to pass. So, unless you are certain of well over 60% of the answers, you must give replies to other questions of which you are not absolutely certain. If you are certain of only a third of the required replies then in order to pass you must mark many questions about which you have at least a minor degree of uncertainty.

7

Oral examinations – including clinicals

'When he who hears does not know what he who speaks means,
and when he who speaks does not himself know what he means,
then chaos reigns.'

Voltaire.

Oral communication is an everyday essential activity of every
practising doctor, and therefore oral examinations which assess
not only the amount of factual knowledge but also the ability to
convey it, must be an important, although never the sole
component, of medical examinations.

The art of any oral examination is to convey an attitude of
confidence and self-assurance, even if not possessed, without on
the other hand appearing to be smug or arrogant. How to exhibit
an air of self-confidence has been discussed in Chapter 4 and all
the advice given there, including how to get on well with the
examiners, applies equally to all oral examination. Unfortunately,
some examiners are even more subjective when conducting and
marking oral examinations than written papers. For all examiners
there must· be an arbitary selection of subjects to be asked, and
each within a limited range within those subjects, because of the
time factor. These defects reflect the biases of the examiners and
can be remedied.

But whereas in any written paper the examiners look for errors
of omission, in an oral they are far more likely to listen for and
note any errors of commission. In other words, to any oral
question you are likely to give an incomplete reply and complete
and perfect answers are rarely expected, but saying something that
is obviously wrong is likely to be noticed and pounced upon by
even a semi-somnambulant examiner. You can undoubtedly
afford some errors of omission in an oral but errors of commission
are likely to have dire consequences.

No silences

'Never remain silent when a word may put things right, for
wisdom shows itself by speech, and a man's education must find
expression in words.'

New English Bible translation of Ecclesiasticus 4:24.

Silences never gain marks, and candidates must realize quickly
that the examiner is waiting for him to talk and he should do so
instantly. In such circumstances many candidates, when they do
finally talk, hedge their answers with expressions indicating
doubts. This is often done and blatantly exhibits a fear of being
wrong which many examiners find maddening.

On the other hand, some candidates are so afraid of giving a
wrong answer that they hesitate unduly before replying to each
question. They should appreciate that such silences are caused by
obsessive fears, and are displays of lack of confidence, be they
engendered by genuine uncertainty or pathological fear of making
a mistake, but they will never help the candidate to gain the
esteem of the examiners, most of whom regard speed of correct
replies as eminently desirable. Your task in any oral is to keep
talking whenever allowed to do so. You must try to prevent the
examiner from dozing.

However, if it appears to you that the silence is due to the
examiner dozing you must realize that you are failing in your
mission to impress him and keep him interested in what you are
saying. You must always endeavour to keep him alert and
attentive. It is not your duty by repeated silences to give any
examiner respite from the possible tedium of listening to
candidates. Your task must always be the continuing and
continuous imparting of information. You must never become
aphasic. Marks are never given for silences whatever the reason
for them. With many candidates such periods are due to a delusion
that by such a practice they will at least make no mistakes, but
neither will they score any marks. Aristotle tells of the philosopher
Cratylus who decided never to say anything except what he knew
to be certain, but as a consequence he ceased to talk at all and
confined himself to wagging a finger.

If the examiner asks you about some subject you have never
heard of or cannot immediately recall, then it is no use maintaining
a stony silence. For example, if asked to talk about erythema
multiforme exudativum and you cannot readily think what that is,
then immediately but politely and appealingly, with appropriate
'sir' or 'madam', and 'please', ask whether that condition has

another name. If he then informed you that it is sometimes called Stevens–Johnson syndrome you may be enlightened and able to talk unhesitatingly. This technique should also be used when asked the use of some drug for which you have been given the proprietary name and you know only the generic name or vice versa. On the other hand, if no help is forthcoming as a result of your request for elucidation, then do not remain crestfallen and dumb or try to put on an act, but acknowledge, without any trace of pride, that you are indeed ignorant on that subject, and look appealingly and hopefully that he will pass on to some other subject.

A common reason for a candidate's silence is because he is thinking of a plan or gathering together his thoughts before committing himself to a reply. But this practice is not productive of marks and, especially if the question is deemed an elementary one, will create a very bad impression. Remember that either you already have a plan which you can follow and give quickly or no plan at all, and in the latter contingency you are extremely unlikely to think of a suitable one at such a time of stress. So, start talking right away and hope further inspiration will come as you proceed.

Some peculiar examiners, however, like to do all the talking, either to show how knowledgeable they think they are, or in a wrong-headed endeavour to teach the candidate, and then you must listen attentively and at appropriate intervals thank him for the information, however irrelevant or even false you may consider it to be.

Elocution

'Open your mouth and let your words be clear.'

Judah ben Bathyri, Talmud Berachot 22a.

I have often thought how much many candidates would gain from a few elementary lessons in elocution. This is especially true of Afro-Asians and others for whom English is a second language. Mumbling, talking with a hand across the mouth or with fingers inside that cavity, or with many 'ums' and 'ers', are all too often great detractors from many candidates' performances. Many examiners get annoyed if they have to ask a candidate to speak up or repeat something. Something said by a candidate but not heard by the examiner is as though it had not been mentioned at all. Clear elocution is often a sign of self-confidence. Moreover, it is most unusual for a candidate to be told that he is talking too loud but many candidates are told to talk louder. So avoid whisperings and mumblings which betray your lack of self-confidence. Indeed, most candidates should talk a little louder than they ordinarily do. If sitting at a table do not hold a conversation in a low voice with the examiner immediately next to you but instead address the examiner furthest away, thus guaranteeing that all examiners will be able to hear you distinctly. To avoid any possible confusion when using the prefix 'hyper-' or 'hypo-' always pronounce 'hyper-' as a long syllable and 'hypo-' as short as possible.

You must also practise and develop an accuracy and fluency of verbal descriptions which are essential for meaningful communication between candidate and questioner. The three Cs – Clarity, Conciseness and Confidence – must always be your aim.

Avoidance of waffling

Always try to get to the gist of any answer as quickly as possible without any preliminary waffling or being sidetracked by some minor issue. For example, if asked the treatment of severe haematemesis do not waste time (which might by justifiable in a written paper) by a detailed preliminary discussion of causes or investigations. A suitable opening gambit would be, 'The commonest cause of haematemesis is a peptic ulcer and, if the diagnosis has definitely or with reasonable certainty been established, I would treat the patient as follows.' Vagueness of thought is associated with vagueness as to the precise meaning of words used, and a lack of clearness of expression indicates a corresponding lack of clearness of thought. This applies not only to oral examinations but also to essay questions. Moreover, it must always be appreciated that many words, both technical and non-technical, may mean different things to different people – for example, secondary optic atrophy – otherwise you and the examiner may be talking at cross purposes.

Never don a Latin or Greek cloak in an attempt to hide your British ignorance. The first essential to clear thinking and speaking in an examination is an ability to quickly recognize with certainty exactly the point of the questions and to stick precisely to the point until it has been dealt with fully to the best of your ability. It is the hallmark of the vague and muddled thinker that he drifts from one point to another, wandering hither and thither without thinking. A clear thinker recognizes quickly what the examiner wants to hear. Some candidates avoid answering the question asked but instead apply themselves to a question that they wished they had been asked. The question should never be repeated or its wording altered.

Imperturbability

You must be prepared to be asked something about which you know very little or even nothing, or the examiner may inform you brusquely that your answer was wholly or partially wrong or irrelevant or inappropriate or reasonable but not what he wanted, but such setbacks must not be regarded as indicating failure. Coolness under all circumstances even when everything appears to be going wrong, and clearness of judgement even at moments of stress, should be your aim. What you must try to develop is an imperturbability, a sang-froid, in the face of such upsets, otherwise your morale will be so shattered that you will go from bad to worse and find yourself saying things which you yourself know are crazy, in reply to subsequent even simple questions. To be prepared for such contingencies is to be forearmed. Never show by your manner, speech or actions any annoyance with any examiner even if you consider he is behaving unreasonably or even unfairly, or talking nonsense.

Many examiners claim that they reserve the very difficult questions, or even impossible ones, for those who have shown by their previous replies that they must be amongst the successful. Unfortunately this is often not so and I could name several examiners who seem to gain a sadistic pleasure in destroying a candidate's morale near the beginning or even at the outset of an oral examination. Such men should never be allowed the honour and privilege of being examiners. Other examiners when challenged to justify their asking peculiar or impossible questions reply that if the candidates do not know the correct answers it is not counted against them. Why then disturb the candidate by asking such questions? Only a conceited examiner asks questions in an examination to which he does not expect a correct answer.

Politeness

You should insert the occasional judiciously placed 'sir' (or 'madam') without appearing to be unduly condescending or grovelling, but as an expression of politeness and an acknowledgement of the relative positions of yourself and the examiner.

Precision of language

'The chief merit of language is clearness and we know that nothing detracts so much from this as unfamiliar terms.'

Galen.

As advised in the chapter on Essay Questions (Chapter 5), whenever a technical word or phrase is first introduced into the conversation it must be immediately defined. The same applies to the mention of any syndrome. Useful bridging phrases are, 'By which I mean, sir,' or, 'Which is characterized by.'

Remember that you personally, by your own answers, determine many of the questions that you are asked because most examiners will ask you to explain and define any terms you use and also demand that you justify any statement that you make.

Too many candidates too readily trot out the latest neologisms and catch-phrases even though they be counterfeit and fraudulent or not understood properly if at all, but when, not surprisingly, they are asked to define those smart-alec words and phrases they miserably fail to do so. An oral examination is not the time to be made suddenly aware of such inabilities. All your words and phrases should be as simple and as non-controversial as possible. Certainly no word or phrase should ever be used which you cannot readily explain and show you understand. It is especially in cardiology that unthinking and uncritical candidates use terms derived from the science of rheology, such as ejection or flow or turbulence, but when challenged to explain those terms they cannot do so. The latest scientific jargon is to be avoided at all costs unless fully understood. So decide before you go into any examination whether you yourself understand such jargon, and, if not, avoid its use unless the examiner himself introduces such terms.

Jargon often adds confusion because it tends to hide rather than explain in spite of its aura of precision. Moreover, often different people using the same term are talking about and considering different things. Technical jargon far from being precise often leads to misunderstandings between candidate and examiners. It is too often mere mumbo-jumbo, making true communication with examiners difficult. Follow Schopenhauer's advice, 'Describe extraordinary things by using ordinary words'. Jargon and the latest neologisms too often make simple things complicated and complex things incomprehensible.

Your definitions must always be precise and in intelligible and logical language and must never contain other technical words or equivocal or controversial phrases or words that themselves require definition or explanation. The use of romantic descriptions, especially those which are far fetched or contain terms with which you yourself are not familiar, must always be avoided unless the examiner obviously demands them. For example, the romantic description of the spleen in lymphadenoma as 'hardbake' should not be used unless you know that this refers to a type of toffee of which you know the special distinctiveness. Unfortunately, two descriptions of certain types of arthritic hand deformities have become popular, especially with those who do not understand the terms or their application, namely, 'swan-neck' and 'boutonnière'. I am amused to discover from some standard medical dictionaries that the latter term which is French for 'button-hole', is still defined medically as the incision made in the penile urethra to remove a calculus.

Medicine is a cliché-ridden subject but you must try to avoid the use of terms that, when correctly used, have a limited and very special connotation, even sometimes a precise diagnostic significance. When discussing many diagnoses what is often required is a flexibility and manoeuvrability, a mentioning of probabilities rather than any certainty. For example, the term 'sabre tibia' is usually taken to imply a definite syphilitic aetiology and is not synonymous with a bowed tibia, the term being derived from a short sword with a forward curvature of its upper half. Similarly, 'tufting of the terminal phalanges' indicates a certain diagnosis of acromegaly, and should not be used unless that is implied.

Avoid eponyms unless specifically asked for them. They are likely to be followed by such absurd questions as: 'Who was X?'; 'Where and when did he live?'; 'What exactly did he describe?'; 'Was it a truly original description?'; and other questions which are likely to be profitless and bring no joy but increasing anxiety and depression. A difficulty is that some examiners demand the frequent use of eponyms and wrongly consider that lack of such knowledge is a grievous fault. A fuller discussion on eponyms is given in *A Primer of Medicine* (1984, 5th edition, Butterworths).

Avoidance of abbreviations

What has been said on this subject in Chapter 5 on Essay Questions, applies with at least equal force to all oral examinations including clinicals. An opening statement such as 'The patient has CCF as shown by JVP plus and also has AF with MS', is likely to be met with scorn and derision by most examiners. Be self-critical long before any examination and try to determine whether this is a fault of yours. If it has become an ingrained habit you may not realize that you are addicted to abbreviations, especially if it is a common practice in your medical school, unless you analyse your own speech habits when talking medicine and decide that you must avoid the vice from now on. Otherwise, during examinations you are certain to fall into this error even though you may be determined beforehand to avoid the practice. Such bad habits are very difficult to correct unless assiduously avoided for at least many months prior to the examination. Moreover, it must be realized that many medical abbreviations are interpreted differently by different people. A fuller discussion of this is given in *A Primer of Medicine.*

Criticism of the examination material

Never even give any hint of criticism of any material that any examiner may show you. Do not comment that any X-ray is not technically good because of over- or under-penetration or incorrect placing of the X-ray tube. Do not demand additional X-rays such as laterals or obliques before you have discussed fully the film that you have been shown. Clinical photographs, however faded or out of focus, or bad colour prints, must never be criticized on any of those accounts.

Also, when shown an electrocardiograph, clinical photograph or positive X-ray do not automatically turn it over to the reverse side, because if the diagnosis is written there, which well it might be, then the examiner will be greatly displeased. You are not likely to do this deliberately, only accidentally, but even so the examiner is likely to be annoyed.

Finally, at the end of any oral examination, including clinicals, before leaving always thank the examiners in a voice that at least sounds sincere. Never, including in clinical examinations, attempt to explain or justify mistakes.

'And oftentimes excusing of a fault
Doth make the fault the worse by the excuse.'
                                        Shakespeare. *King John,* Act 4 scene 2.

8

Clinical examinations – general remarks

'The ear that hears, the eye that sees.'

Proverbs 20:12.

Preparation

Reading must play an important role when preparing for medical examinations but clinical ability, the art and science of dealing with patients, is never proportional to the amount of time spent reading. On the contrary reading, especially uncritical, may turn any student into a learned fool and a bad clinician. Moreover a great difficulty, especially for undergraduates and recent graduates, is the ability to make a correct assessment of the calibre, experience and actual honesty of some of the contributors to medical journals.

The main preparation for any clinical examination should always be examining as many patients as possible during your years of clinical study. Unfortunately, nowadays, final qualifying examinations and even postgraduate degrees and diplomas are often overconcerned with biochemistry and mathematical data, which information can be learned and understood without the benefit of genuine clinical experience or an ability to elicit and interpret clinical signs properly. In many medical schools students are repeatedly exhorted to spend more and more time in medical libraries. But this is not the way to become a competent physician. Clinical ability cannot be achieved by spending most of your time reading.

Instruments

Although some instruments, and sometimes all necessary ones, are usually provided it is far better that you bring your own. Rushing around a ward to borrow some instrument wastes time which may be very precious. If the borrowed instrument is of poor quality, for example, a torch or ophthalmoscope light may be inadequate, you cannot complain and you have no redress. You should have with you instruments that are old familiars and with which you are used to working. Take with you the following instruments, unless otherwise stated.

Stethoscope

The stethoscope must have both bell and diaphragm. Neither the earpieces nor the bell must be cracked, chipped or broken. The earpieces must be correctly angled and fit without discomfort and the rubber tubing must be thick, inelastic, and rigid so that the two lengths do not collide and rub against one another causing artefacts. The bore of the tubes should be about 5 mm and their length about 15 cm. Never borrow a stethoscope especially for an examination or buy a new one only a few days before, lest you be unfamiliar with that stethoscope's idiosyncrasies, and auditory hallucinations bombard your ears and cause confusion. When buying a stethoscope it is mandatory that you are discriminating in your choice and do not buy a model merely because it has become fashionable; buy one that suits you personally.

Tendon-reflex hammer

Small light hammers, which are very popular, have the advantage of easy portability but are not satisfactory. They will not produce an adequate stimulus unless used with a fair amount of force, so that if an examiner asks you to demonstrate tendon reflexes, you may have, or at east appear to have, to use considerable vigour, especially if the reflexes are sluggish, and this may produce adverse criticism from the examiner. A good reflex hammer is fairly heavy with its main weight in the head, has a long cane or plastic handle and is well balanced. It must be held far away from its head so that it describes as large an arc as possible before it reaches its point of impact. It is this extent of movement that makes any undue force unnecessary.

Torch

There are many suitable pocket torches on the market. It must produce a strong narrow light beam. I strongly recommend that you buy new batteries for it a day or two before the examination.

Old batteries which appear to be adequate have a bad habit of failing you at a critical time.

Tape measure

You probably will not have reason to need this but it takes up very little room and its use at an appropriate time may gain you some valuable additional marks, for example, measuring chest expansion, rather than recording it as poor; measurement of head circumference when suspecting a congenital hydrocephalus; measurement of the girth of a limb when muscle wasting is diagnosed; or measuring limb length as an indication of joint dislocation or lack of growth. Expressing such facts in figures often impresses examiners.

Pin and cottonwool

Have these kept in a convenient readily accessible place.

Tuning-fork

Entirely different forks are required for testing defects of hearing and for vibration sense. Good and worthwhile tuning-forks are, at least in Britain, very expensive because they are unnecessarily accurate for a physician's use, so that if it is labelled a C256 it is precisely that. This is because in Britain they are not made primarily for neurological examinations but for singers and testing musical instruments. You may not consider it worth your while to buy one of each type especially for an examination and this may be a reasonable judgement. In the latter case you will have to rely on the correct type of fork being available but this is sometimes not the case as many hospitals are badly equipped in this respect.

Thermometer

This is another instrument which is well worth taking in with you even though you are unlikely to find need for it. But when examining a patient as a long case with respiratory infection or rheumatoid arthritis, or a patient with a heart lesion in whom you suspect bacterial endocarditis, pointing out to the examiner that you have taken the temperature and found it raised may get you a few extra marks.

Spatula

Two or three wooden spatulae take up little room and may be useful. Having your own spatulae handy may prevent wasting precious minutes seeking for one.

Ophthalmoscope

It is no use borrowing an ophthalmoscope with which you are not familiar, even if it is the most expensive type. You must have an instrument that you yourself have frequently used. It is stupid to use, for example, a wide-angle instrument in a clinical examination if you have never or rarely used one before. As with a torch, buy new batteries a few days before the actual examination.

Sphygmomanometer

Because of the bulk of most of these instruments I do not suggest taking one in with you. When shown a heart lesion as a short case it is extremely unlikely that you will have time to record the blood pressure or be allowed to do so. For a long cardiovascular case you should have ample time to find and borrow a ward instrument.

Carrying your instruments

It is often preferable for men not to bother with a carrying case at all but instead to put as many instruments as possible in various pockets, knowing exactly where each is and from which each can be readily retrieved. This may well leave only an ophthalmoscope and possibly a reflex hammer to carry. Briefcases and the like can be a nuisance and many candidates appear to be at a loss what to do with them when being questioned by examiners. Other candidates waste time and get flustered rummaging in their case for the required instrument.

Female students are at some disadvantage in not having so many pockets, and some examiners would look askance at any women who produce a required instrument from some hidden recess. But be careful in the selection of an instrument bag. It must look reasonably professional, of subdued colours and not psychedelically embellished. It must have various compartments so that there is not the slightest difficulty in finding any wanted instrument quickly. Such a bag should contain the barest minimum of personal non-medical effects. Shopping-bags or baskets are never suitable.

Preliminaries

You are certain to be shepherded into the ward where the examination is held by a junior member of the staff who is helping the examiners. It is essential that you ask him how long you will be allowed for the long case. It would be silly to complain to any examiner that you had had insufficient time unless you were in a position to tell him that you had had far less than you had been personally informed you would be allowed. You must also ask that junior doctor if a specimen of urine is available because if it is then this is proof that you will be expected to test it and you must allow time to do this. If it is a women's ward you must ask about nurse chaperones. Also enquire from where any instruments may be borrowed that you have not brought with you. Even if you have met that junior doctor before, and even if you know him personally, do not embarrass him by seeking any diagnostic help from him or any favours; for example, do not implore him to take you to a patient who has a particular system involved or even hint at some preference.

Any clinical examination can be discussed under two headings: (1) the candidate's relations with the patients; (2) the candidate's relations with the examiners. God forbid that British teachers and examiners should ape the Americans by employing professional actors to play the part of patients and simulate special diseases, or showing slides or cine-films instead of actual patients. May we be saved from a new generation of students prodding plastic swellings in dummies and analysing artificial urine. Our profession must be protected from technomaniacs who consider clinical medicine to be a game which can be played with artificial materials instead of actual patients, and that by manipulating a computer, even a badly programmed one, clinical ability can either be learned or assessed.

9

The long case – history-taking

History-taking is a major diagnostic procedure often of no less importance than physical examination, and each must be considered as essential complements one to the other. The greater the skill in obtaining a history the more reliable and extensive will be the facts on which a diagnosis is later based. Moreover, history is more than just questioning and listening but should be accompanied by careful observation of the patient.

To obtain a satisfactory history in the limited time at your disposal it is essential that, right from the onset, you must try to get on good terms with the patient. You should begin by introducing yourself and telling the patient not only your name but also where you come from. Shaking hands with patients is not to test their grip or degree of perspiration but as a greeting to a fellow human being. Your approach must be continually friendly, sympathetic, warm, kindly, generous, good mannered and humble, and never arrogant, blown out with an air of feigned superiority.

It is essential to learn from the patient as quickly as possible his main symptom or symptoms which motivated him to seek medical advice. Concerning each individual symptom enquiry must be made about its duration (which need not be known exactly); its mode of onset; how it has subsequently progressed; all possible factors, including treatment, which may have relieved or aggravated it. If pain is a leading symptom then its site, radiation, nature severity, frequency, and aggravating and relieving factors must be elucidated. It is imperative that you do not allow the patient to skip from one symptom to others before you have obtained a full account of each individually.

Always be aware that the examination time is limited and time is fleeting. So, the length of time spent on history-taking is important and at all costs you must avoid the common error of spending too much time on this. You are unlikely to be successful if you miss some important clinical findings and this is likely to occur if you do not leave yourself adequate time for detailed examination of the patient. You must always assume that there is at least the possibility that every system is affected and so every system must be examined carefully, but if you have spent too long on the history there will not be enough time for that.

The actual length of time spent on history-taking must depend on the total time allowed for the long case. If that total time is 45 minutes then history must occupy at most 10 minutes, and if the time allowed is 60 minutes then the time spent on the history must be at most 15 minutes. But getting a history and doing a physical examination should always be regarded as a continuous process and never as two completely distinct and entirely different activities. So, after you have completed the examination it may become obvious and imperative that you must ask further details of history. For example, you should not as a routine ask every patient about his alcohol consumption because, for one thing, you may find yourself wasting time trying to assess such phrases as, 'not really heavy', or 'only moderate' or 'only the same as my workmates', etc. On the other hand, if on physical examination you discovered that the patient had peripheral neuritis or an enlarged liver, then it would be essential to go back after completion of the physical examination and make the appropriate enquiries. To give another example, details concerning an attack in childhood or adolescence of 'rheumatism' would be mandatory if you later found evidence of heart disease, but such details would be of no value and the time spent in obtaining them wasted if the patient is found to have syringomyelia without any coincidental heart lesion. This same advice applies to social history, which is usually irrelevant, although it may occasionally be of importance. Moreover, if family history and previous illnesses are enquired into at great length before details of the main complaint have been elaborated the patient is likely to get bored or irritated which will militate against a good doctor–patient relationship which you should be trying to establish. There are a few examiners who invariably demand precise details of social history and all previous illnesses and family history regardless of any possible relevance to the diagnostic or therapeutic problems involved. Such examiners are guilty of intellectual dishonesty because they are usually purposely or subconsciously wasting time so as to avoid full discussion of the real condition about which they know very little or even nothing. I know of one examiner who spent most of the allotted time asking all candidates about diabetes regardless of the patient's actual condition. Against such manoeuvres candidates are helpless.

Some patients, if you allow them, may waste a good deal of your time, often albeit with the best of intentions and with a genuine desire to help. But be on your guard against such misplaced zeal or loquacity. You must politely and subtly steer the patient towards more practical information and along channels likely to be more profitable to you as a candidate. To give an example, a woman who complains of sudden onset of paralysis of her legs may, if you allow her, go into great details about the person with whom she was at the time, or in which shop window they were gazing, and what they were nattering about when the blow struck. Or another patient with a similar history may stupefy you, if you do not intervene, with a verbose but completely irrelevant account of her belching dyspepsia. You must at all such times make a rapid decision as to whether the information being supplied is likely to be relevant. Remember that after completion of the physical examination you may realize that your assessment that some particular symptom was unimportant was in fact wrong, but then you can go back and obtain further details. If a patient cannot remember an exact date do not let him waste time by reference to his diary or let him struggle trying to recall the precise time. In such cases always insist that you want only an approximation. Do not let the patient waste time with such details as the names and addresses of the various doctors he has consulted and the hospitals he has attended.

The commonly given advice that you should allow patients to tell their story in their own way and in their own time with little or no interruption is impracticable and bad advice when applied to any clinical examination. With some patients, in the time allowed you would not complete even the history let alone the physical examination as well. Careful guiding and polite interruptions are usually essential. Some leading questions which provoke the patient to give one type of answer rather than another, or a definite instead of a vague reply, may quickly yield important information. If the patient is deaf, or has a very poor memory, or has only a very rudimentary knowledge of English, do not despair and do not waste time trying to obtain the unobtainable within the limited time at your disposal; for example, by writing your questions if the patient is deaf. Such patients are likely to have many positive physical signs and the sooner you start searching for them the better.

When you have completed the volunteered history always then ask some essential leading questions, for example, concerning appetite, bowels, weight and micturition, if any of these topics have not been previously mentioned. In other patients other leading questions are often necessary; for example, in a patient with a neurological lesion, concerning disturbance of vision (including double vision), headache, attacks of loss of consciousness and disturbances of micturition. Such essential questions for each individual system should have been taught to you and clinical experience should have emphasized their relative importance.

In conclusion, remember and always be aware of the fact that incomplete physical examination is a common cause of failure and a frequent reason for that is spending too much time on the history.

10

The long case – physical examination

Before the actual physical examination of the patient you cannot ever be certain which systems are affected. For example, a patient complaining of cough and expectoration may not only have a lesion of his respiratory system but may, for example, also have splenomegaly and a neurological lesion, either of which may be related or unrelated to the chest condition. Moreover, the patient may not have even hinted at such additional lesions, possibly because he himself is genuinely unaware of their presence. In other words, all systems must be examined in all long cases and it must never be assumed that any system is normal because the patient has not volunteered any referable symptoms.

The comparative difficulty of each of the long cases should be as equivalent as is reasonably possible. Unfortunately, a strong tendency has developed to show some long cases with very few or even no positive physical signs. This often leads to bad examining, encouraging some examiners to waffle themselves or allow candidates to do so unchecked, or to devote most of the time to theoretical or obscure aspects of medicine, or to matters that have little or even no relevance to that particular patient. Some examiners seem to ignore the fact that a clinical examination should deal with clinical matters.

It is more than likely, whether the examination is a qualifying one or for a higher diploma or degree, that you will be asked to demonstrate the positive physical signs and how you sought for those that are not present. This task is likely to be accomplished satisfactorily only if you have spent much time and trouble during the months and years of your preparation for the examination in attempting to perfect those techniques. Physical signs cannot be mastered by reading books but only by their repeated performance on many patients. It is not my intention in this book to describe the eliciting and interpretation of physical signs, because these important matters are described in detail in *A Primer of Medicine* (1984, 5th edition, Butterworths). When eliciting signs, meticulous attention to the precise details of each technique is crucial. The good candidate must be concerned primarily in any clinical examination with the methods of seeking for signs and the logical interpretation of findings, negative and positive. Boasting of knowledge of trivia and minutiae and the latest theories and such academic waffle can never be a substitute for genuine clinical ability. The budding violinist concentrates on technique and avoids consideration of such academic nonsense as to whether he is playing on a logarithmic scale. The golfer who wishes to improve does not waffle about the physics of trajectories or aspects of elasticity, but concentrates on improving his techniques and correcting any faults. So it should be with you in regard to clinical medicine.

Order of examination of the long case

When examining a long case always do so from above downwards and do not automatically start with the part of the anatomy about which the patient is complaining. This means examination in the following order: head and face (including cranial nerves), mouth (and related structures), neck, upper limbs, heart, breasts, lungs, abdomen and lower limbs. The reason for this is to avoid the necessity of the patient having to dress and undress repeatedly throughout the examination. For example, do not examine the cranial nerves, then the upper limbs from a neurological viewpoint, the abdominal reflexes, and later a detailed neurological examination of the lower limbs, and then go back to examine the other systems. There is no valid objection and many advantages in examining the various parts of the body from above downwards rather than confining your attention to each system one at a time. What you must avoid is leaving any patient completely or semi-nude: for example, when looking at the lower limbs leaving the upper part of his body uncovered because you have not yet examined the heart or lungs. The patient may resent such a practice even if guarded by screens or curtains and such a disregard for patients' feelings is likely to produce a lack of the desirable help and co-operation which you want from every patient. Also the patient may complain about your conduct to an examiner, perhaps with disastrous consequences to yourself.

If the patient is a female any chaperone will insist that as you proceed from one part of the patient to another you reclothe the parts not being examined. Repeated dressing and undressing will waste time. I recall an incident when I was helping with a final MB examination for which the late Sir Arthur Hall was the senior external examiner. He drew my attention to a happening at the other end of the ward and asked me to investigate. A female candidate was examining a stark-naked man who was attempting to perform the heel and knee test as an indication of ataxia. There were no curtains or screens around the bed. When I remonstrated with her the candidate replied that she did not think it was in the least important because the patient was blind. Sir Arthur Hall was not amused, or at least did not show it, and admonished the candidate, much to her disquietude and chagrin. Professor Hall of Sheffield was the finest examiner whom I have ever heard and from him I learned a lot about the art of questioning to assess people's knowledge and ability. He was not only a distinguished neurologist but also a good general physician and excellent dermatologist and held successively three different professorships – those of physiology, pathology and clinical medicine. He was a truly complete physician, the like of whom we shall probably never see again. One of my own teachers, the late Lord Cohen of Birkenhead, also deserves a place in this select pantheon.

Avoidance of hurting patients

Never hurt patients. The examiner is likely to hear their cry of pain or protest, or the patient may issue an ultimatum that he does not wish to take any further part in the proceedings, and when the examiner enquires the reason he may be told that the candidate hurt him in some way. On such occasions, and usually with justification, the examiner will be prejudiced against the candidate. No candidate would deliberately hurt any patient but is likely to do so if his techniques of examination are bad, or he persists with some procedure such as eliciting plantar reflexes again and again in a futile attempt to overcome his indecision. Do not leave a bleeding patient caused by overenthusiastic but ill-considered energy when testing pain sensation. Do not leave scratch marks caused by that same procedure. To attempt to elicit abdominal reflexes with a sharp instrument is disgraceful even if you may have seen some consultant neurologist do that. When later you are asked to demonstrate those reflexes your stupid and thoughtless action will become manifest and will cost you dearly.

A valuable 5–10 minutes

With the long case you must always leave sufficient time, at least 5 minutes, so that after completion of the ordinary physical examination you will have ample opportunity for the following:

1. To test urine if it is available.
2. If the patient has a neurological condition to test for Rombergism and gait if he is able to walk.
3. To examine the spine if there is any suspicion that this might be involved, either because of other joint involvement or the finding of a focal lesion of the spinal chord. The only satisfactory way of examining the spine is with the patient out of bed and standing if able to do so.
4. After you have completed the physical examination and any of the above three procedures, but never before, you must always leave adequate time to ask the patient the following questions:

   (a) What is the diagnosis? It can nearly always be readily assessed whether or not the patient really knows.

   (b) What investigations have been done and what did they show? Here also it will almost invariably be easy to assess whether the patient is giving you accurate information. This enquiry is of great importance because you are certain to be asked which investigations you yourself would advise, and it will obviously be judicious to enumerate those to which the patient has been submitted, without of course mentioning that the patient has given you this information. The patient's information may be very rewarding. For example, if you have considered that this cardiac irregularity is due to extrasystoles but he informs you that an electrocardiograph showed fibrillation, then it should force you to reconsider your verdict and realize that you are probably wrong. No patient will ever deliberately mislead you on such matters. Moreover, the nature of the investigations that have been done may give valuable clues as to either the actual diagnosis or along which lines the consultant in charge of that patient is thinking if no final diagnosis has yet been made. For example, in a patient with a spastic paraplegia who has had a myelogram this would indicate that the probability of cord compression is at least being considered.

   (c) What treatment has the patient had and with what results? You are certain to be asked for your suggested treatment and the most sensible answer would be to suggest the therapy that the patient has actually received unless it has produced definite deleterious effects. Do not boast that the patient has given you this information. If, for example, the patient has rheumatoid arthritis and is on steroid therapy, or the patient has a mild degree of hypertension and is on hypotensive drugs, or a patient with a valvular lesion is scheduled for surgery, do not even hint, whatever your actual views, that such therapy is not advisable.

(d) Always ask the 'long case' if he knows what questions are being asked about him and the replies that the examiners expect. You will probably not get any help here but it is always possible that you could obtain some surprising information which may be your salvation. For example, the patient may inform you that the examiners are interested in a neck swelling and want to know if it is expansile or not, when, in fact, you may not have discovered such a swelling. Any actual demonstration of physical signs will vary in one important aspect according to whether (i) you have been asked to demonstrate a particular sign justifying your diagnosis of a particular lesion, for example, chest percussion as evidence of an effusion; or a limited group of signs supporting a diagnosis, for example, of ascites, or a cerebellar lesion; or (ii) if asked to examine the whole or part of a system, for example, cranial nerves, or part of the body, for example, the lower limbs. In the former event you should demonstrate only the positive physical signs but must be prepared to answer the very likely follow-up question, namely, 'What other (or confirmatory) signs did you look for?'. Your reply should be immediate without any hesitations, listing all the other physical signs of that particular lesion which you sought but found not to be present. For example, having said that the patient has a pyramidal lesion of both lower limbs, you then demonstrate the positive signs you found, for example, extensor plantar reflexes, increase of some or all tendon reflexes, and weakness of some or all muscle groups of the lower limbs. When later asked for other evidence you had looked for, you then list the other signs, spasticity (which you define) and clonus. Anticipation of that second question should ensure that when you examine patients you always look for all the described signs of any particular lesion and not be content at finding only one or a few of them. The sin of greed must be avoided.

On the other hand, if the examiner has asked you to examine some part of the body while he observes your techniques, you must recite all your positive and negative findings whilst you continue to examine the patient, explaining what you are seeking and with what result, and this must be done in the classic order, inspection, palpation, percussion and auscultation, whenever appropriate.

5. Finally, and often most important, always leave yourself at least 3 minutes during which you will carefully consider how you intend to present the history, the physical signs, the diagnosis and its differential, and what questions you are likely to be asked and how you intend to answer them. No candidate can afford not to spend adequate time in this preparation before the examiners pounce on him with their initial questions. It is often asking too much of yourself to expect to be able to work all this out satisfactorily whilst you are actually being questioned. To be prepared before the examiners tackle you may be the key to your success.

The long case – presentation of history

Always try to make your recitation of the patient's history as concise as possible and devoid of all irrelevancies. Some examiners delight in grasping any and every opportunity of avoiding questioning on the actual diseased condition. For example, if the patient has syringomyelia avoid giving the examiner irrelevant information such as, that the patients's mother had diabetes or the patient himself had diphtheria when a child. There are unfortunately some examiners whose knowledge of clinical medicine is so specialized and even very limited that they are incapable of spending the whole time allotted for genuine discussion of the particular patient's actual condition, but try at the slightest opportunity to get on to their own pet subject, which is very unlikely to be to the candidate's advantage. So, do not deliberately give any information which you know is completely irrelevant to the particular patient's diagnosis, investigation or treatment, just because you have obtained such information from the patient. Even with a neurological case of long duration it is usually possible to give a satisfactory history in a very few words, such as: 'Mr. Smith, aged 65, has had difficulty in walking for 5 years, which came on very gradually and has slowly got worse without remission. He has no other symptoms. And, on examination I found. . .'.

Of course, the examiner may intervene and ask for further details, even irrelevant ones, but then you must obey his wishes. There must be no hiatus between completion of your pithy history and the detailing of the signs, as this will give some examiners their opportunity to ask irrelevancies concerning the history. It is your account and discussion of physical signs which are much more likely to get you good marks, so the sooner you describe those findings the better.

The long case – general remarks on presentation of signs

'There is no more difficult art to acquire in medicine than that of observation and for some it is also quite as difficult to record observations in brief and plain language'.

Sir William Osler.

Never start with a minor, unimportant or irrelevant finding. For example, having examined a patient with a neurological lesion do not start with an irrelevant skin lesion. At all times, but especially used as an opening gambit, avoid vague indefinable phrases such as 'The patient has a sallow complexion' or 'The patient's nutrition is inadequate'. The examiner's first questions are likely to be centred on explanations of such a finding or phrase, probably to your great discomfiture.

Always start with the system primarily affected. If more than one system is involved and you have doubts as to which is primary, or more or most important, then always start with the system about which you feel most confident concerning both the signs you have found and their interpretation.

Diagnoses

Diagnoses should always be discussed from defined and acceptable premises to a clear conclusion. Correct premises are an essential prequisite of any type of logical reasoning, and never more so that when considering a diagnosis. Moreover, the more reliable the evidence the more valid will be the inferences derived from it. Beware of making what has become some recently fashionable diagnosis, which often is really a cloak of ignorance.

Diagnoses must always be considered in stages and in the great majority of patients the first-stage diagnosis is an anatomical one; stage two should be in terms of general pathology; and stage three your considered opinion as to the certain, probable or possible final diagnosis stated in terms of some special cause of the general pathology cited. As an example, having been asked to examine an abdomen and then asked the diagnosis, your initial answer must always be in anatomical terms, for instance, 'This patient has splenomegaly'. You should follow this by your reasons why you considered the swelling to be a spleen and not, for example, a renal enlargement. Your second-stage diagnosis should then give the most probable general pathology causing that patient's splenomegaly, for example, a blood disease such as —; or a reticulosis such as —; or an infection such as —; or associated with hepatic cirrhosis (portal or biliary, according to the evidence). Your final diagnosis should be the most likely cause, in that particular patient, of each general pathology. Another example, having examined a patient's nervous system and found pyramidal lesions of the lower limbs, your answer to the question, 'What is the diagnosis?' should be the first-stage, the anatomical diagnosis, for example, 'He has a pyramidal lesion of his lower limbs as shown by . . . '. Whenever possible, state the definite or probable site of the lesion within either peripheral nerves, spinal cord or brain. Your second-stage diagnosis should be in terms of general pathology, for example, a degenarative lesion such as X. The third-stage diagnosis depends mainly on the history, which with short cases you would not know. Moreover, it must be realized that with many patients, and especially with the short cases, the first-stage, that is the anatomical diagnosis is the only one that can be made with certainty and the other two diagnostic stages can be discussed logically only in terms of probabilities and, later, of possibilities. But there must be no misunderstanding on this matter. To say that, for example, a patient has hepatomegaly or an extrapyramidal lesion is a diagnosis, albeit only a first-stage one. You must avoid the bad habit of questioning the examiner as to what he personally means by the word 'diagnosis'. You must never indulge in the slightest quibbling on this issue and must be very firm in your own mind concerning the notion of stages of diagnosis. On the other hand, if the question asked is 'What is the complete (final) diagnosis?' you must not hesitate to give a third-stage diagnosis immediately, either as a certainty or probability according to the weight of the observed evidence.

Presentation of the individual systems

The best way to present any case is the way the examiner expects and wants, but obviously you do not know his wishes and possible personal idiosyncrasies and it would never be advisable to ask him outright how he wants you to present the case. The methods which I advise have been very carefully thought out for many years and have yielded many successes. Many candidates and unfortunately many examiners have never seriously considered the pros and cons of the numerous possible methods of presenting various types of cases.

Speed of answers

Speed of replying to all questions is of prime importance. Hesitation always indicates a lack of self-confidence and uncertainty. Many questions demand a quick and simple reply, often either a 'yes' or 'no'. Hesitancies and ditherings are hallmarks of lack of self-confidence. Delays at such times may make the examiner jump to the conclusion that you are guessing, even if this is not true. For example, if asked, 'Has the patient got mitral stenosis?', if there is an interval of many seconds before replying, or of your answer is not a simple 'yes' or 'no', many examiners will suspect, either rightly or wrongly, that you are guessing or not sure. On the other hand, replying with alacrity and conviction may hide your indecision and get you marks which, in fact, you may not deserve.

An examiner who was noted as a bully grew impatient with an Asian candidate and bawled, 'Answer me, yes or no. Has the patient got mitral stenosis?'. The candidate edged very close to the examiner and, in a whisper, answered, 'perhaps'.

No waffling (see also Chapter 7, page 45)

Never indulge in preliminary waffling before actually answering. For example, after having felt a patient's abdomen, when asked for findings do not start with some such completely unnecessary verbiage such as, 'On examination of this elderly man's abdomen on palpation I found an enlarged spleen'. Instead of such verbosity answer immediately, 'This man has splenomegaly'. Another example is that when some candidates are asked for their findings in a heart case they start off with some opening remark as, 'On palpation I felt a thrill and on auscultation I heard a systolic bruit'. How else could anybody discover a thrill except on palpation or a bruit other than on auscultation? Heed the advice given by Ben Sira in Ecclesiasticus (Chapter 20, verse 8), 'He who uses many words shall be abhorred'.

A further example of waffling – when asked to listen to a patient talking, the bad candidate advertises his ignorance by answering questions in the following vague ways:

Candidate: 'This patient is difficult to understand.'
Examiner: 'Why?'
Candidate: 'Because he has a speech defect.'
Examiner: 'What type of speech defect?'
Candidate: 'A scanning speech.' (Incidentally, this is a term often used incorrectly and inappropriately.)
Examiner: 'What is the technical word to describe such defects?'
Candidate: 'I do not know any other term.'
Examiner: 'Would you say that he has dysarthria?'
Candidate: 'Yes, perhaps.' ('Perhaps' is a word often unnecessarily added by many candidates when under stress. It betrays a complete lack of self-confidence.)
Examiner: 'And what is the cause of the dysarthria?'
Candidate: 'Multiple sclerosis.' (This appears to be the only neurological condition known to some candidates and is too often mentioned wrongly as the most probable diagnosis.)

Presented with such a problem the good candidate immediately replies 'Sir, he has dysarthria'. And when questioned about the cause, gives a quick answer, such as 'An extra-pyramidal lesion because he has a coarse compound tremor of the limbs'. If the examiner has to drag information out of the candidate by repeated questioning, especially when a simple answer to the initial question was all that was required, then the marks awarded are likely to be very few indeed. Moreover, such a performance often irritates examiners and causes them to lose their patience and become testy, petulant and hypercritical.

Do not repeat the examiner's questions

With many candidates this is a pernicious habit of which they are themselves unaware, but many examiners are likely to show displeasure if every question is automatically repeated. Worst of all is to repeat the question with an air of incredulity or, by your intonation, suggest that you consider the question to be a stupid one. For example:

Candidate: 'This patient has nystagmus.'
Examiner: 'What kind of nystagmus?'
Candidate: (in an aggressive or petulant manner, perhaps with facial contortions indicating annoyance): 'What kind of nystagmus?'

'I think'

Never, when giving physical signs or a diagnosis, use the phrase 'I think', either at the commencement or at the end of your remarks. For example:

Examiner: 'Has the patient mitral stenosis?'
Candidate: 'I think she has mitral stenosis', or 'She has mitral stenosis, I think.'

Such unnecessary use of the phrase is likely to be interpreted as lack of certainty.

Notes

With the long case you should make at least brief notes on history and signs but do not refer to those notes when talking to the examiners.

Facetiousness

Never be facetious or attempt 'judicial humour' or levity, as they are likely to backfire.

Abbreviations

Avoid colloquialisms and abbreviations

Confessions

Many candidates exhibit a peculiar habit of behaving as if they were in a confessional, asking forgiveness for their sins of commission and omission. Never mention, let alone boast, of what you have inadvertently or purposely not done. Never confess to having found a sign difficult to elicit unless you have a good excuse for that difficulty. For example, never mention difficulty in determining the position of an apex beat unless you know a justifiable reason for this (such as gross emphysema), or boast that you had difficulty in visualizing fundi, without giving an adequate reason (such as small pupils). Above all, never admit having forgotten to do something essential, such as recording the blood pressure. Always conceal your mistakes and your difficulties and hope that you will not be found out.

The short cases – general remarks

'The trouble with doctors is not that they do not know enough but that they do not see enough.'

Sir Dominic Corrigan (1802–1880).

Information obtained by sight, hearing and touch are nearly always reliable guides to diagnosis provided that it is fully appreciated that hallucinations and illusions may occur, and also that the interpretation of the significance of any definitely positive signs may be wrong. Certainly more is missed by not looking carefully than for any other reason. The eyes used as wide-angle lenses are for most people more reliable evidence than the ears. The usual time allowed for each short case is about 5 minutes except in those cases where a complete diagnosis is possible on inspection alone, when only a minute or two is likely to be allowed. The candidate must never assume that he will be given more than 5 minutes for any short case unless otherwise told. Speed, especially in getting to the right wavelength immediately, is often the essence of the task.

Short cases are often 'spots', that is, of a type that should be readily recognized on inspection. Dermatological and joint and endocrine lesions often come within this category. The candidate is expected to get on to the correct 'wavelength' and to state the diagnosis immediately. This may well be a final one, such as psoriasis, gout, or acromegaly, or a first-stage diagnosis, such as bilateral ptosis or bowing of tibia or exophthalmos.

Other short cases often shown are eyes (including fundi), deformities of the hands due to various causes and lesions of heart, lungs, abdomen, or cranial nerves. Examination and the differential diagnosis of all of these are discussed fully in *A Primer of Medicine*.

Reasons for failure

Many candidates who regard themselves as at least competent clinicians often have great difficulty with the short cases. Candidates often find themselves under great stress for which they are neither prepared nor accustomed. Much of this stress arises from the limited time allowed and the fact that the examiners are often watching critically, perhaps making the candidate acutely and embarrassingly aware of his shortcomings. But it is stupid and of no value to object to how any particular examination is conducted. You must be prepared for and graciously conform with the procedures imposed upon you. For example, it is of no use to maintain that your cardiological ability is at least adequate if allowed 15 minutes to examine a heart, when in fact you are allowed only 5 minutes. The ability to perform and assess speedily all procedures must be frequently and diligently practised long before the actual examination.

Sometimes the examiner does not inform the candidate precisely which system to examine; for example, he may ask him to look at the lower limbs. This is another common cause of failure with the short cases, because the candidate does not get on to the correct wavelength quickly and the usual cause of this failure is because he does not properly use his eyes, those God-given wide-angle lenses. Many, shown a patient with parkinsonism, will fail to notice the diagnostic tremor and suggest some completely different diagnosis, perhaps not even neurological. A candidate asked to examine hands may fail to notice the joint swellings and discuss neurological instead of arthritic conditions. Of all the physical signs anywhere in the body those most commonly missed completely are those which should have been found by inspection alone. Auscultatory failures are not, as so many candidates have been led to believe, a common cause of lack of success in clinical examinations. Moreover, it must be realized that when the candidate is on a completely wrong diagnostic wavelength the examiners often do not correct him but instead discuss the condition wrongly diagnosed, and even if the candidate does this well he is unlikely to be rewarded with many marks.

You must always try to anticipate the likely questions concerning the physical signs and think of the answers while you are actually examining the patient, instead of guessing them when you are questioned. For example, with any heart case you are almost certain to be asked three fundamental questions, namely, rhythm, heart size, and a full description of any bruits. These then must be always your prime consideration when examining any heart. Another example is that if you have found that a patient has arthritis you must anticipate the questions: 1. Why arthritis and not, for example, a neurological lesion? 2. What is the nature of the arthritis? Another example is that if asked to examine the lower limbs and you notice bowing of one or both legs then you should anticipate that you will be asked (a) its certain or probable cause; (b) the differential diagnosis; (c) justification for your preference. To be impressive your answers must always be speedy, logical, relevant and valid, given with an air of confidence.

Another common reason for failing on the short cases is that many candidates indulge in wild guessing, and, when challenged to give valid reasons to support their diagnosis, they realize too late that they cannot. If you do this once and you are later allowed to retract and make a more sensible or reasonable suggestion, you may possibly be excused, but if you continue with your wrong notions then the certain outcome will be failure. This attitude to clinical medicine arises from and is perpetuated by the fact that most of those who indulge in this type of diagnostic guessing are uncritical of themselves and are often even oblivious that this is one of their own major faults. Instead they prefer to bask in the sunshine of that one occasion when they guessed correctly and made what appeared to be a brilliant diagnosis. They forget that their guesses were almost invariably not only wrong but very wide of the mark and rarely correct. Students should be taught that they must be able to justify each and every statement they utter.

If asked to examine, for example, the neck and the candidate sees what appears to be an enlarged thyroid he must be prepared to give the evidence on which he based that diagnosis, namely, site of the swelling and that it moves with deglutition. He should then examine the thyroid swelling carefully in the traditional order of inspection, palpation and auscultation, including feeling for enlarged cervical lymph nodes and the position of the trachea and any evidence of retrosternal extension. Very important, he must complete his diligent search for positive and negative findings in the thyroid itself before looking for exophthalmos, associated eye signs, tremor or sweating, or evidence of myxoedema.

A discussion differentiating the procedures required when asked to demonstrate a single sign or a limited number of signs compared with if asked to demonstrate the signs in the whole or part of a clinical system or part of the body, for example, the limbs, is given at the end of Chapter 10.

With the short cases I strongly recommend careful attention to the following.

(1) *When the examiner asks you to look or listen to some part of a patient,* for example, the heart, it should always be assumed that a full examination of that particular part of the body is required, unless the examiner specifically asks you to listen only, or inspect only, etc.

(2) *Do not talk to the short cases* unless specifically asked to do so, except to ask those essential questions which really form part of the physical examination, such as when palpating an abdomen to enquire concerning local tenderness, or when examining ocular movements to question the patient concerning any history of double vision. To enquire about matters such as previous illnesses or even symptoms is nearly always a waste of precious time. To ask the patient the diagnosis is inadvisable as you and the patient are likely to be overheard by the examiners.

(3) *Examine immediately the system you have been asked to examine* – For example, if it is the heart do not examine either the abdomen or the lung bases, or look for oedema at ankles or sacrum, or listen for a bruit over the femoral arteries, until you have completed in detail the examination of the heart itself, which must include the pulse and observation of the neck (*see A Primer of Medicine*). Otherwise you may be interrupted and asked about your findings in the heart long before you have completed the actual examination, having devoted most of the time to extra-cardiac signs. If you have completed the actual heart examination and you still have further time before questioned then you should seek out the other signs mentioned, but usually you will not have sufficient time to do so.

(4) *A request to examine the chest* should always be interpreted as meaning the respiratory system unless definitely told otherwise by the examiner.

(5) *When examining limbs from the neurological point of view* always first complete the motor system aspects (power, wasting, tone, reflexes and co-ordination with eyes open and closed) before doing any sensory tests. This is advised because in the majority of such patients the motor abnormalities are more important than the sensory, .and are more likely to be present in the absence of the other and not vice versa; moreover, you are often not allowed sufficient time to do both carefully.

(6) *It is prime importance that you assess all physical signs with speed* – and, if in doubt whether a particular finding is present, such as tracheal deviation or cardiac enlargement, or optic atrophy, it is always advisable to describe the suspected abnormality as not present rather than base a diagnosis on a doubtful finding. For example, whether a patient has clubbing can be and must be judged in a second, and prolonged staring and holding the fingers in various positions and stroking the nails is of no avail but is merely time wasting and a betrayal of lack of confidence.

Moreover, to conclude and later inform the examiner that some sign is slightly positive, such as clubbing or tracheal deviation, is usually either an expression of profound conceit or lack of confidence. The significance of a slightly positive sign is nearly always the same as if that sign were markedly positive. The causes of sluggish ankle jerks are the same as the causes of absent ankle jerks; the causes of minor degrees of tracheal shift are the same as those of marked deviations; the causes of sluggish pupillary reactions are the same as those causing complete absence; the causes of a slight accentuation of any heart sound are the same as those that produce a marked increase, etc.

The truth is that many, even when not battling in examinations, use the word 'slight' as a spurious insurance cover against later being accused of missing something. Such people commonly use other words and phrases for the different systems that have the same significance as the word 'slight'. For example, they claim, without the faintest trace of boasting, that they have heard a very soft short systolic bruit, or seen a minor degree of pallor of a limited part of the optic nerve, or that the lower margin of the liver was 'just' palpable, or that they have 'tipped' the spleen. I am reminded of the princess in the fairy story who claimed the remarkable ability of being able to diagnose the cause of her disturbed sleep as a single pea hidden beneath 20 mattresses piled one above the other. A claim to be able to 'tip' the spleen is typical of this uncritical attitude and the word 'tip' may be appropriate, conjuring up as it does, impressions of gambling, hunches and guessing. Unfortunately with many medicals such descriptions become an automatic performance, giving the perpetrator a subconscious escape from the necessary task of confident and unequivocal decision making as to whether any supposed finding is truly present. If you cannot definitely see, feel or hear something then your attitude should be that you have not seen, felt or heard what you had attempted to see, feel or hear. This rule applies, of course, equally to the long as well as the short cases.

(7) *Do not expect the examiner to inform you that you are either right or wrong* – A 'yes' or a nod or shake of the head does not indicate that you are either right or wrong. With many examiners saying 'yes' or nodding is a tic or a manoeuvre to keep themselves awake. Because of this many candidates come out of a clinical believing that they have done well when in fact they have failed. When they have diagnosed mitral stenosis, rheumatoid arthritis and diabetic retinitis in each of three consecutive patients and the examiner has said, 'yes' perhaps several times and with slow definite nods, they incorrectly assumed that lack of contradiction

signified agreement. No examiner is ever under an obligation to tell you when you are wrong or to give you an opportunity to correct any mistakes. Most examiners stop their questioning and go on to the next case either because you are correct or obviously wrong. A few examiners unfortunately play a cat-and-mouse game and ask questions about any positive signs that the candidate claims to have discovered, whether right or wrong or even of no relevance. This happens most often with heart cases; for example, if a candidate diagnoses heart block instead of atrial fibrillation with a slow ventricular rate he may be asked a series of questions concerning heart block, even if the examiner knows that that diagnosis is wrong.

(8) *If you have been asked to examine only a limited part of a patient* – for example, his lower limbs or hands – you must not assume that he has or has not any positive signs elsewhere. It is quite likely that you will not have time to examine another part of that patient. On the other hand it is considered to be fair by most examiners to expect you to have observed some other part of the body which is readily accessible to inspection. For example, if asked to look at the lower limbs and you have found arthritis of ankles or knees it would be very reasonable to expect you to glance at the hands, because if they are arthritic the variety is usually most readily determined there rather than at other joints, and also absence of arthritis of hands makes the diagnosis of rheumatoid extremely unlikely. Moreover, it should take only a few seconds to make this assessment. Another example is that if asked to look at the hands of a middle-aged man and they exhibit arthritis, the glancing at the ears for tophi would probably be expected. A further example is that if a middle-aged or older person has aortic regurgitation without any other valvular disease you should glance at the face to see if bilateral ptosis with frontalis overaction is present, and, if there is sufficient time, whether the pupils are abnormal.

Sometimes the showing of only a limited part of the patient is very unfair but the candidate must not complain. This often happens with dermatological lesions, the examiner not appreciating the importance of distribution as an essential diagnostic guide and also that over the part of the body shown the rash may not be typical. Examples of this are:

1. Expecting the candidate to diagnose neurofibromatosis with certainty when he has not been allowed to look at the patient's trunk for the café au lait zones which are invariably present there and not on limbs or face.

2. Expecting the candidate to readily recognize as psoriasis an atypical area over the abdomen, or when elbows and knees showing typical lesions are not readily available for inspection.

These and many other possible examples are due to the examiner's ignorance and not his perversity or sadism.

Many examiners adopt a good policy of asking the candidates to look at X and anything else the candidate may consider to be important diagnostically. Obviously, the 'anything else' depends on the assessment of X and if that is wrong it is very unlikely that 'the anything else' you choose to examine will be helpful. For example, if asked to examine the lower limbs and 'anything else you like' you are unlikely to look for exophthalmos and diplopia unless you have correctly diagnosed pretibial myxoedema. Another example is, if asked to look at the hands and anything else, you would not think of examining the ears for tophi unless you thought the hand abnormality was probably or possibly due to gout.

(9) *Be careful that you never accidentally hurt a patient* – For example, by clumsily grabbing her arthritic hands, or too frequent and too enthusiastic attempts to elicit plantar reflexes.

(10) *Ideally, when the examiner has finished asking about a particular patient and then takes you to the next case* you should try to forget immediately any difficulties or contretemps about that or any previous patient. Many start examining a new case still worrying about the previous mistakes and difficulties, and rethinking replies to former questions. Rather, be like a good professional tennis player who immediately forgets the error he has just made and concentrates on winning the next point. The whole art of success in clinical examinations consists in always concentrating all efforts on the one point or points immediately at issue. Stephen Zweig wrote (*World of Yesterday* (1943), page 149): 'The eternal secret of all great art, yes, of every mortal achievement, is concentration'.

(11) *When you have finished examining each individual patient* – Thank him or her and on no account leave the patient half-naked.

(12) *Always sprinkle your conversation* at appropriate intervals with 'sir' ('madam', if the examiner is a woman). This must not be overdone or sound obsequious or patronizing, but if judiciously spaced will let the examiner know that you appreciate and are aware of and unhesitatingly accept your relative positions.

(13) *When you are dismissed by your examiners* – Thank them in a voice that at least sounds sincere.

14

Presentation of physical signs in abdominal cases

When asked to look at or feel an abdomen you must always assume, unless distinctly told otherwise, that a detailed examination of the abdomen is necessary and not merely inspection or palpation. When examining an abdomen never neglect to glance at the conjunctival mucous membrane and the genitalia (in a male patient) and feel for enlarged lymph nodes and look for hernias.

Whether the exact wording of the examiner's question is, 'What have you found?' or 'What is the diagnosis?' or 'What is the matter with the patient?' you must always start, 'Sir, this patient has . . .' and give the abnormality you have found in precise anatomical terms such as, an enlarged left kidney, or a colonic swelling, or an enlarged bladder, etc. You should then immediately give your reasons why you consider the swelling to be anatomically what you stated it was. You must give these signs without hesitation and nothing should be dragged out of you. Often you would have been unable to elicit all the expected signs of that particular enlargement; for example, you may not have felt a notch in an enlarged spleen or been unable to feel above an enlarged kidney. In such cases you must always be prepared for the question, 'What other signs of an enlarged X did you look for?' Again, your answer must be unhesitating and to the point.

Many examiners have the good habit of asking each candidate to draw a diagram of what they have found, so you must be prepared for this and be certain that when you palpate any swelling you seek out all its details, including its exact site, shape and size and which borders are well defined and if its surface is smooth or irregular, all of which points can be accurately represented on a diagram. Correct appreciation of those details can be achieved only by examining every abdomen with great care and concentration.

If the patient has more than one swelling in his abdomen you should present these one at a time, starting with the one that you consider to be the more or most important diagnostically. For example, if a patient has an enlarged spleen and liver do not present the case as one of hepato-splenomegaly or as hepato-megaly but start with the enlarged spleen and mention the hepatomegaly only after you have described the splenomegaly. This is because in patients with both of those organs enlarged it is the splenomegaly that determines the order of your differential diagnosis, and makes the diagnosis of secondary or primary hepatic malignancy unlikely, whereas that would be a strong possibility even if not a probability if only the liver were enlarged. Furthermore, this method also avoids the dangers of trying to discuss two things at the same time and causing confusions and misunderstandings, because either you or the examiner is not clear exactly which of the enlargements you are discussing at any particular moment.

If you have been asked to examine the abdomen and you have observed some significant extra-abdominal findings, such as arthritis of the hands, do not mention this until after you have described the abdominal findings. If relevant you must mention the extra-abdominal sign or signs when you are discussing the second-stage and third-stage diagnosis.

You may be asked to demonstrate the physical signs and this is especially likely if you have diagnosed ascites. So, before you make any such suggestion, remember that you will be challenged to demonstrate the signs. For example, in the case of ascites this would especially be the marked dullness in both flanks, and if you have any doubt about your ability to demonstrate this in that particular patient, then the diagnosis of ascites should not be made.

15

Presentation of signs in respiratory cases

Unless told to the contrary, when asked to 'look at' or 'listen to' a chest you must always assume that a full examination of the respiratory system is required. This must always include the position of the apex beat, and looking for clubbing, cyanosis and enlarged lymph nodes in neck and axillae, and examining the breasts.

When presenting your findings you must always start with a first-stage diagnosis, which should be a statement of the general pathology (effusion, pneumothorax, consolidation, collapse, or fibrosis), combined with giving the exact site and extent of the lesion. With the exception of bronchitis and/or emphysema never diagnose more than one pathology at the same site, for example, collapse and consolidation of the same lobe. Of course, two such pathologies may occur at the same site but it must be emphasized that on physical signs alone it is nearly always impossible to be certain of this because the physical signs will be of one lesion only. However, with a long case the history may yield good evidence of an additional pathology at the same site. For example, in a patient who has signs of collapse of a lobe, a history of mucopurulent sputum would be strong evidence of infection (consolidation) of that lobe secondary to the collapse.

The physical signs can, and always should be, given in as few words as possible, devoid of introductory waffle, repetitions, and negative findings. For example, a good opening gambit, when appropriate, would be, 'Sir, this patient has fibrosis of the right upper lobe as shown by impaired movement, percussion and breath sounds all over that area and there is flattening of the chest and deviation of the trachea'. Do not waste time repeating the signs anteriorly and posteriorly if these are identical. Avoid waffling tautological phrases such as, 'On percussion there is dullness and on auscultation there is an area of bronchial breathing'. How else could dullness or bronchial breathing be found except by percussion and auscultation, respectively?

After stating the first-stage diagnosis and your valid reasons for this you should then proceed to discuss the probable final diagnosis, namely the cause of the effusion or collapse or whatever your first-stage diagnosis was. In a long case it may be possible, but only very occasionally, especially from details of the history, to give a complete diagnosis with certainty and justifiably be able to use the phrase, 'The patient has . . .?'. But even with long cases this is often not possible, sometimes not even with a high degree of probability. With short cases, lacking a clinical history, it very rarely is possible to make a certain complete diagnosis and so this must be discussed in terms of probabilities and later of possibilities. Stated differently, with short cases it is rarely justified to state, 'This patient has got (for example) cancer of the bronchus'. Such a presentation indicates an irrefutable certainty which is usually born of either conceit or ignorance. Moreover, if you make such an unjustifiable definite final diagnosis it is likely that the examiner will not bother to contradict you or ask for an alternative opinion but will demand the reasons for coming to such a definitive conclusion. By further questions he may indicate indirectly, if you will but listen and retract, that your reasons are not sound.

You are very likely to be asked to demonstrate the physical signs and you should be able to do this with supreme confidence. It is percussion that frequently is very badly performed, the candidate often proclaiming to the examiner by repeating the performance again and again over the same area that he is very unsure of his findings and he may even betray this further by going back and repercussing an area over which he has just auscultated. Each successive percussion over the same area is likely to produce a different note because of involuntary variation of technique with each stroke, striking the pleximeter finger at different angles each time or with varying intensity, or varying the period during which the pleximeter finger is pressed on the chest, or bringing your ears nearer and nearer the patient with each successive percussion. For full discussion of this and other techniques the reader is referred to *A Primer of Medicine*. Moreover, in your anxiety, increased by the examiner's careful scrutiny, you may forget to percuss the axillae or feel for trachea or lymph nodes. By repeated practice and with radiological checks you should become confident of your ability to elicit physical signs correctly long before you enter for any clinical examination.

Often a temperature chart is purposely left at either the foot of or above the bed and this should be looked at quickly. If a sputum mug is left on the bedside locker its contents should be observed. Both of these observations should take only a few seconds.

16

Presentation of signs in neurological cases

Whenever possible try to comply precisely with the following.

(1) *Always present the signs* in terms of stages in diagnosis, the first an anatomical one, naming the sites of each lesion one at a time. For example, 'Sir, this patient has a right third nerve lesion as shown by . . ., and pyramidal lesions of both lower limbs shown by . . .'.

Never start with an isolated sign such as a dilated pupil or sluggish ankle jerks, or extensor plantar response. A presentation such as, 'Sir, this patient has bilateral cerebellar signs as shown by . . .' is far better than starting, for example, 'Sir, the patient has nystagmus', and then being quizzed as to the type of nystagmus and its significance. My suggested methods shows self-confidence but the second type of approach is likely to result in a very unconvincing display, everything being dragged out of you by a barrage of questions. Another example, it is far better to start by stating that the patient has a pyramidal lesion of the lower limbs as shown by an extensor plantar response and listing any confirmatory evidence and the other signs sought for but found to be absent, rather than beginning, 'This patient has an extensor plantar reflex'. Moreover, adherence to my suggested method should act as a constant reminder when you are examining each patient that every physical sign has a probable or certain localizing value but never gives a definite clue to the likely pathology. For example, nystagmus does not indicate disseminated sclerosis but may be very good evidence of a cerebellar lesion or its connections, provided that you can demonstrate supporting signs.

After giving an anatomical lesion and the reasons why, do not alter the technique of presentation by then mentioning some unrelated physical sign or signs before stating the anatomical site of a second or third lesion which has produced the additional signs not explainable by the first anatomical lesion diagnosed. For example, having said that the patient has pyramidal signs in both lower limbs and giving the evidence for that, do not then switch tactics and mention that, for example, the ankle jerks are sluggish, but decide beforehand the reason in anatomical terms for the sluggish reflexes, such as a lower motor neurone lesion as shown by wasting of the calf muscles in addition to the sluggish ankle jerks; or a posterior column lesion as shown by diminution of joint and/or vibration sense and ataxia with the eyes closed in addition to the sluggish ankle reflexes. Again, emphasis must be made that often not all signs, which may occur as a result of a lesion in a particular site, are always present and that the sin of greed must be avoided.

(2) *The physical signs elicited must be stated without hesitation and with an air of confidence* – Statements such as, 'There may be slight pallor of the optic disc' are to be avoided.

(3) *Having given the signs that led you to make each individual anatomical lesion* you must always be prepared for the questions, 'What other physical signs of that lesion did you find?' And if your answer is 'None', then you must anticipate that you will be asked for a list of other physical signs which you should have sought. Lack of promptness of all replies to these questions is likely to cost you dearly. There are but few possible signs of each individual lesion, so there can be no excuse for forgetting even a single one; for example, clonus as a sign of a pyramidal lesion.

(4) *Be precise with each anatomical lesion* – So that when mentioning, for example, a pyramidal lesion immediately state which limb or limbs are affected and, when diagnosing a lower motor neurone lesion, mention which muscles are affected as shown by focal wasting. (Always be prepared to demonstrate the appropriate wasting which is a fundamental sign of any lower motor neurone lesion of limbs, neck muscles, or tongue.)

(5) *When, as is common, more than one part of the nervous system is involved* – Always start with the cerebral cortex if it is affected and give the reasons for this localization. Then, one by one, give the cranial nerve lesions if any and your reasons for the diagnosis. Then mention, one by one, any long tracts that are involved and name the parts of the body affected and the physical signs you elicited to support each diagnosis. Finally, enumerate any motor and/or sensory peripheral nerves involved. Again it must be emphasized that each lesion should be given singly and the positive physical signs recited immediately. Never attempt to describe the physical signs of two lesions at the same time, for example, cerebellar and posterior column, as this is certain to cause confusion and misunderstandings.

(6) *Never initially recite a list of negative or normal findings* because by so doing you would be merely wasting time without gaining any marks. On the other hand, as stated previously, the

examiner may later ask which if any of other expected signs are present and he may ask you to demonstrate how you sought for them.

(7) *Having given each lesion and the reasons for each* – You should then attempt to place all the lesions in a single anatomical site. For example, if the patient has a right third nerve lesion and a left upper motor neurone hemiplegia you must point out that these two lesions together indicate disease of the right crus cerebri. Another example is that if the patient has a lower motor neurone lesion of his hands and an upper motor neurone lesion of his lower limbs, these two findings point to disease of the spinal cord at the level of the first thoracic segment.

(8) *You may be asked to demonstrate the signs* – And in that case, after mentioning each lesion individually and in the order suggested (note 5), instead of reciting the signs you must demonstrate them. Make sure that you really know how to elicit neurological signs in a convincing way and indicating that you have done this often before and are fully conversant with the orthodox techniques (*see A Primer of Medicine*). It must be realized that there are several reliable ways of eliciting individual physical signs, for example, ankle jerks, plantar responses, or ataxia, and the candidate should be aware of some of those other methods. Examiners, especially those who are not neurologists, may disapprove of your method but in that case you must be prepared to change your technique without explanation or justification of why you used your initial method, and do so without displaying any annoyance or reluctance to change.

(9) *The second diagnostic stage* is in terms of general pathology and this will usually depend primarily on the history, especially the precise mode of onset and subsequent progress of the condition. With short cases, lacking a history, the second-stage diagnosis cannot be given with certainty except in a few instances; for example, in the presence of Argyll Robertson pupils. Therefore, in the short cases you should immediately give a differential diagnosis without any preliminary shilly-shallying, but starting with the most probable final diagnosis and if asked the lesions that you might find in parts of the body that you have not examined.

(10) *When asked in the long case for the final (complete) diagnosis* – Always commence with the one that you feel is either certain or most probable. If the patient has told you the complete diagnosis, always start with this, without of course telling the examiner that you have been so informed, and do not attempt some misguided gamesmanship by first giving one or two

deliberately wrong diagnoses in a futile attempt to hide the fact, which anyway the examiner probably knows, that the patient has given you all the correct information.

(11) *When asked for a differential diagnosis of any neurological case,* short or long, always discuss disseminated sclerosis, neurosyphilis, spinal cord compression (if there is a focal cord lesion), and brain tumour or cerebral vascular lesion if the signs are localized to the brain. After mentioning each suggested alternative diagnosis you must give valid reasons why you did not consider that condition more probable than your final choice. In other words, you must always consider not only your reasons for making a diagnosis but also each and every piece of evidence against any other diagnosis. You should try to quantify any adverse evidence in terms of whether it definitely rules out that diagnosis or makes it probably or possibly less certain. Such an attitude must always lead you to think of alternatives in any case where the final diagnosis is not certain. Any unusual features should make you self-critical and cast doubt on your apparent certainty. Many wrong diagnoses are due to boasting that you know that in a small percentage of cases such and such a finding is unusual but does occasionally occur.

Presentation of signs in cardiovascular cases

Never start with negative findings such as absence of cardiac failure, or jugular vein distension or clubbing or cyanosis, etc. Such a recital wastes precious time without gaining marks. Moreover, in a short case you can never be certain that cardiac failure is absent, not having obtained a history of, for example, dyspnoea on exertion, and not having examined the patient completely. It would be embarrassing if you said that a patient has not got cardiac failure and then, when asked to look at the sacral area, you find gross oedema and are forced to contradict your previous opinion. Start with cardiac failure if the evidence is beyond doubt and you are fully aware that no single sign such as cyanosis or jugular vein distension, or even both together, is not pathognomonic.

Mention any signs that you may have noticed outside the heart itself only when present beyond doubt. Never, when uncertain, attempt a bogus insurance against missing anything by claiming some particular sign was 'slightly' present or of minimal degree, for example, clubbing, cyanosis or a bruit. Moreover, having mentioned that some sign was 'slightly' positive you will be challenged to demonstrate it and to state its significance and possible causes, and your replies will have to be prompt and unhesitating if they are to carry conviction.

Having described any relevant positive extra-cardiac signs you should then state the rhythm in concise and technical language, such as atrial fibrillation or atrio-ventricular block, and never in vague terms such as, 'The heart is irregular'. Do not use the terms bradycardia or tachycardia because by themselves without qualification they lack precision and their mention is likely to provoke silly quibbling as to what exactly numerically constitues a tachycardia or bradycardia. If the rate is definitely abnormally slow or abnormally fast state that rate as determined by counting with a watch over a 10-second period. In the short cases you cannot afford to count the pulse rate for a longer period, but it must be appreciated you would not fail because you said that the rate was 64 when the examiner's record stated it was 56, or if you said that it was 90 when it was actually 100. But you would lose marks if your estimation was well out and this is likely if you do not use a watch.

An authentic account of a candidate's time-wasting performance is as follows:

Candidate: 'The patient has a bradycardia.'
Examiner: 'What do you mean by a bradycardia?'
Candidate: 'A slow heart.'
Examiner: 'How slow.'
Candidate: 'There is no generally accepted figure.'
Examiner: 'Would you describe a rate of 64 as a bradycardia?'
Candidate: 'No Sir.'
Examiner: 'Does 62 constitute a bradycardia?'
Candidate: 'No Sir.'
Examiner: 'Does 60?'
Candidate: 'No Sir.'
Examiner: 'What about 58?'
Candidate: 'It may do so, Sir.'
Examiner: 'So your definition is a rate of 58 or less?' (The candidate became increasingly disturbed by what he wrongly considered to be quibbling by the examiner.)
Examiner: 'What is the cause of this patient's slow rate?'
Candidate: 'It may be a sinus bradycardia.'
Examiner: 'Due to what?'
Candidate: 'The patient may be a marathon runner or recently recovered from typhoid.' (The examiner's obvious incredulity at the mention of these two conditions upset the candidate even more.)
Examiner: 'Go back to the patient and count his pulse rate.' (The candidate was further embarrassed when the examiner discovered that the candidate did not have a watch and had to borrow the examiner's.)
Candidate: 'The rate is only 46.'
Examiner: 'Now what do you think?'
Candidate: 'He may have heart block.'
Examiner: 'What type?'
Candidate: 'Complete.'
Examiner: 'So, do you now think that he has got complete heart block?'
Candidate: 'Yes Sir.'
Examiner: 'What further evidence would you look for?'
Candidate: 'Cannon waves.'

Examiner: 'Has the patient got them and, if so, will you demonstrate them?' (The candidate could not do so, although he claimed that he had seen them; this was followed by a barrage of questions about cannon waves, their special characteristics, the mechanism of their production and their differentiation from giant 'a' waves. By which time the candidate was completely demoralized.)

In such a case a good candidate would start his initial reply by stating that the patient has complete atrio-ventricular heart block because his heart rate is only 46 and does not increase with exercise (admittedly not vigorous). When answering a question about confirmatory signs his replies would be quick and, when challenged to demonstrate them, he could and would do so convincingly, including stating with confidence that some expected confirmatory signs, which he named, were not present.

The reasons for always starting your account of a heart case with the rhythm are as follows:

1. You are certain to be asked the rhythm; forewarned, therefore, you must always make its determination your first and one of your principal concerns.
2. Many candidates often forget to tell the examiner about a significant arrhythmia, especially atrial fibrillation, even though he has found that, and the examiner may wrongly consider that the candidate has missed it, and not give him an opportunity to mention it later.
3. When a valve lesion has been diagnosed and the examiner then enquires if any other lesion is present, many candidates wrongly consider that they are being asked about other valvular lesions, forgetting that a significant arrhythmia may reasonably be described as a heart lesion.
4. Many patients have an arrhythmia such as atrial fibrillation or heart block without any valvular lesion and in such cases some candidates are always tempted to guess the presence of a non-existent valve disease.

Valvular lesions

After stating the rhythm precisely you should then name any valvular lesion which you consider to be definitely present, and for this part of your presentation I strongly recommend that you adhere strictly to the following rules, unless the examiner demands otherwise.

Rule 1

If you have heard a diastolic bruit of any character you must immediately make up your mind whether it is due to mitral stenosis or aortic regurgitation, or, but far less likely, pulmonary regurgitation, or, even less likely, organic tricuspid disease. (The last named should never be diagnosed as the main lesion or even suggested as a probability in the absence of mitral stenosis.) After having made up your mind quickly as to the definite cause of the diastolic bruit which you heard you should state that lesion (nearly always either mitral stenosis or aortic regurgitation) immediately after you have given the rhythm. Then, having mentioned that valvular lesion, you should state your reasons, preferably with an introductory phrase such as, 'as shown by'. Your first reason must always be a full description of the bruit on which you based your diagnosis, and this description must be complete and in conventional terms (*see A Primer of Medicine*). Many candidates lose marks by having some of the features of the bruit dragged out of them instead of volunteering description of its relative loudness, quality, radiation, thrill, and alterations in its character produced by positioning, respiration and exercise.

Rule 2

The next likely examiner's demand is for confirmatory signs, such as cardiac enlargement or a large volume pulse, and here a common error is mentioning their presence but being unable to demonstrate them when called upon to do so. Remember that not every patient with aortic regurgitation has a collapsing pulse or every patient with mitral stenosis a tapping apex beat or a loud first sound or an opening snap.

Invention of physical signs when they are not actually present is just as blameworthy as missing signs that are present. Moreover, absence of an expected confirmatory sign may have an important significance; for example, aortic regurgitation in the absence of a collapsing pulse would indicate that that lesion is not of severe degree.

Rule 3

The next most likely question is, 'What other bruits are present?' You must then always first describe in full any other diastolic bruit if present, in addition to the one previously described, before mentioning any systolic bruit. The second diastolic bruit must have different qualities from the one first described before you can assume it has a definite different diagnostic significance. For example, if you have presented the case as one of atrial fibrillation with mitral stenosis and given your reasons and you are then asked if you have heard any other bruits, you should then describe the blowing diastolic bruit and all its features if you have heard this. Your account is then likely to be followed by being asked the significance of that bruit, to which your reply would be that it probably (or definitely) indicates aortic regurgitation, for which you will be asked the supporting evidence, if any. Your reply to the last question may well be, if correct, that there were no confirmatory signs. The examiner is then likely to challenge you as to any other possible significance of the bruit. In reply, you should mention functional pulmonary regurgitation secondary to pulmonary hypertension. You will be asked for the supporting evidence for this which you had sought and either did or did not find.

An alternative example is, having diagnosed aortic regurgitation and described the cardinal sign of that lesion (the diastolic bruit of special quality) and the confirmatory signs, if any, you are then asked if the patient has another lesion (or bruit). If you have also heard a rough rumbling diastolic bruit localized to the apical lesion, your reply should be that the patient probably has mitral stenosis in addition to the aortic regurgitation, and you describe your evidence for this. You will then probably be asked for another possible explanation of that diastolic bruit and your reply should be that it may be an Austin Flint murmur and you should discuss the pros and cons of this. Later still, you should describe and discuss the significance of any systolic bruit or bruits.

Rule 4

When the probable or possible presence of another lesion is based on hearing a systolic bruit in addition to the initially described diastolic and you are asked if the patient has another lesion (instead of the more usual question of whether the patient has other bruits), the tactic should be to reply, 'Sir the patient may have . . . (for example, aortic stenosis or mitral regurgitation) because he has a systolic bruit (which you then describe fully)'. Some examiners object when they ask if another lesion is present if the candidate immediately describes a bruit instead of first postulating a lesion and may inform the candidate that a bruit is not a lesion. You must be prepared for such quibbles and immediately alter your terminology so as to satisfy the examiner.

Rule 5

Not only must diastolic bruits always be described and discussed before systolic but a diastolic bruit must never be dismissed as of no significance. A systolic bruit may or may not be significant diagnostically.

A patient may have aortic stenosis and regurgitation or mitral stenosis and regurgitation but the wise candidate presents such a case as either mitral stenosis or aortic regurgitation, and only later discusses the probability or possibility of the additional lesion. Stated differently, in many patients with definite aortic regurgitation the important point of the exercise in a clinical examination is a reasoned discussion of the probable and possible causes of a basal systolic bruit and it is often the logic and thoroughness of your discussion that determines your marks.

Rule 6

Always present one lesion at a time and never two simultaneously. To start by informing the examiner that a patient has aortic regurgitation and aortic stenosis or mitral stenosis and mitral regurgitation or mitral stenosis and aortic regurgitation is always bad tactics, and to start by reciting simultaneously three lesions is foolish. This rule applies even to those cases with definitely multiple lesions and in whom diastolic and systolic bruits can be heard over the whole or greater part of the praecordium. The good candidate describes and discusses each diastolic bruit separately and then, but only later, each systolic bruit.

If the patient has for certainty or probability both mitral stenosis and aortic regurgitation the problem arises as to which one of these to start with, because you should never present two lesions at once. This is but very rarely as big a quandary as it is sometimes made out to be. If the patient is fibrillating, then mitral stenosis must be mentioned first, provided of course that the appropriate bruit has been heard. In such a patient, after having described the signs of mitral stenosis, you should later discuss the probability or possibility of aortic regurgitation also being present and in addition discuss other possible or probable significance of the blowing diastolic bruit, especially functional pulmonary regurgitation. Only after this should you describe in detail and discuss any systolic bruit or bruits that are present.

On the other hand, in such a patient with two different types of diastolic bruit who is not fibrillating and has a large volume pulse, then you must start with the aortic regurgitation describing the appropriate bruit and the supporting evidence. This is later followed by a discussion of the probability or possibility that the patient has mitral stenosis as well (provided that you have heard a rough rumbling diastolic bruit localized to the apical region). Then any systolic bruits are mentioned and described in detail and their definite, probable or possible significance discussed individually.

But if in such a patient not only is the rhythm but also the pulse volume normal, then start with mitral stenosis, mentioning the typical bruit and any supporting evidence. This is followed by a discussion as to whether the patient probably or possibly has in addition aortic regurgitation. Description and discussions of any systolic bruit or bruits again is left till later.

One of the reasons why there is often confusion concerning the techniques of presenting a case who has multiple valvular lesions is because of the use of the term 'dominant' or the term 'main' by either the examiner or the candidate. What you should assess primarily is which is the more or the most important lesion diagnostically and only consider comparative severities of the individual lesions later. The correctness of your diagnosis of the individual lesions is always of greater importance than consideration of any presumed degree of severity, because the correctness of the diagnosis of each and every valvular lesion usually determines definite or probable aetiology of the cardiac condition.

Rule 7

As described fully in *A Primer of Medicine* your description of all bruits must be in simple and conventional terms, avoiding romantic language such as 'seagull bruit', or the language of music or the jargon of rheology (the physics of flow).

Unfortunately it has become fashionable to use the jargon of rheology and to prattle about ejection bruits and of turbulence, laminar or jet types. It all sounds very learned but it is a stupid habit, at least in examinations, unless you are prepared to define these terms precisely, to differentiate between them and explain them in simple language. If you cannot honestly and readily do so then their use will bring trouble on your head because you are very likely to be asked for definitions and explanations. Moreover, the use of these words implies a conceit, a certainty concerning the exact and differing mechanisms of the production of each of these types of bruit. Do you really understand the haemodynamics of normal and abnormal blood flow, including the complex physical laws and formulae involved? Why risk the examiner challenging you on these points and bombarding you with a series of questions on haemodynamics? If the examiner is really an expert on such matters you run the risk that his questions will be beyond your knowledge or comprehension. On the other hand, if the examiner has, as is more than likely, only a confused and confusing smattering of knowledge concerning this most difficult subject, then you are likely to be talking at cross-purposes and it will probably be a case of the blind leading the blind. To describe a certain type of systolic bruit as 'ejection' has the virtue of brevity but this is too often obtained at the expense of a genuine understanding and shows a lack of humility and self-criticism, both essential qualities for a good candidate.

Rule 8

If the patient has a systolic bruit or bruits but no diastolic bruit then the following rules are advised:

First – If there is definite clubbing, cyanosis, increase of jugular venous pressure of orthopnoea they should be mentioned first but negative findings should not be tabulated.

Second – Give the rhythm precisely.

Third – Give the positive signs in the pulse including the rhythm. Do not enumerate the negative findings. Often this necessitates the confident statement that the pulse is normal.

Fourth – Describe the heart size as normal or enlarged. If you consider the heart to be enlarged you must give your reasons for this opinion. If you have experienced difficulty in determining the position of the apex beat, say so, but then you must be prepared to give a good reason why this was so in the particular patient examined rather than a list of possible explanations. For example, it would be stupid to give emphysema as the explanation unless you could demonstrate signs to support this. Describe the apex beat's position and quality in conventional orthodox terms (*see A Primer of Medicine*). Avoid the terms 'hypertrophy' and 'dilatation' because you will have great difficulty in defending the use of one term rather than the other, and it is extremely doubtful that such a distinction can actually be made clinically, especially when there is an element of both, which is often the case. The term 'cardiac enlargement' is always preferable. Do not suggest that the enlargement is 'slight', because this indicates either a conceit that you can clinically make such a diagnosis with certainty or that you are hedging, unable to decide whether the heart is really enlarged.

Fifth – Describe the systolic bruit in great detail, leaving none of its features unrecorded. If there are definitely two different systolic bruits, for example, one loud and long and the other much shorter in duration and possibly different in quality, or when a systolic bruit has been heard over the whole of the praecordium and probably beyond that area, then always first describe the systolic bruit heard at the base of the heart and discuss the probable and possible causes of this in detail before describing the systolic bruit heard in the apical region and probably conducted towards the axilla, pointing out that this other systolic bruit is either a different one to that heard at the base or the latter radiated to the apex and outwards. The reason for advising that the basal systolic be discussed first is that its cause usually determines the most probable cause of the other systolic bruit. For example, if you have come to the conclusion that the basal systolic bruit is certainly or probably due to aortic stenosis then a systolic bruit heard at the apex and possibly conducted outwards is likely to be due either to a functional mitral incompetence secondary to a left ventricular enlargement or conduction of the basal murmur to the apex and beyond. An important fact is that basal systolic bruits are often conducted downwards but apical systolic bruits are very rarely conducted upwards, so, for example, mitral regurgitation alone would not be a satisfactory explanation of a systolic bruit heard over the whole of the praecordium or one heard down the left border of the sternum and apical area. The presence or absence of a thrill should always be regarded as a feature of any bruit and should always be included in its description. Mention of a thrill is often inadvertently forgotten by those who waste time prefacing their description of the signs by the entirely unnecessary phrase 'on palpation there is a thrill'.

Do not attempt to grade systolic bruits numerically, such as 4/6 instead of using less conceited but just as accurate terms such as 'soft' or 'loud'.

Reserve the terms 'functional' and 'organic' for differentiating two types of a valvular lesion and not as a description of a systolic bruit. The terms 'significant' and 'non-significant' are, on the other hand, valuable terms to differentiate the aetiology of a systolic bruit. One of the worst possible presentations of a patient with a systolic but no diastolic bruit is to start with the bruit instead of first stating that the pulse, carotid artery and jugular vein, the rhythm and heart size are normal, or, if they are not, describing any abnormality present, and giving all these facts before mentioning the details of the systolic bruit.

Sixth – Leave any description of heart sounds till the last and then be careful not to boast of your auscultatory prowess, such as hearing summation gallops or paradoxical splitting of second sound.

Seventh – In any patient with a systolic but no diastolic bruit it is rarely possible to give a certain diagnosis, such as aortic stenosis or mitral regurgitation, unless the bruit is completely typical and the supporting evidence (usually size of heart and pulse volume) are also present. In other words, it is not justifiable in such a case to start with a certain diagnosis. Similarly, when asked to give your opinion as to the cause and significance of any systolic bruit which you have described, never start with a certain diagnosis but preface your reply, 'It is probably due to . . .'. What is necessary in most such cases is a reasoned differential diagnosis starting with probability, later mentioning less likely possibilities.

After giving what you consider to be the most probable cause of the systolic bruit, and, if challenged, justifying that opinion, you should then mention one by one all other possibilities, and why you consider each to be only a possibility rather than a probability. No systolic bruit should ever be dismissed as of no significance until after you have discussed all possible causes and the positive and negative evidence against each alternative.

Eighth – A rapid decision must always be made whether to discuss congenital or acquired lesions first. If you do start with a congenital lesion you must be able to give a sound reason for that choice, such as that you have noticed that the patient has some congenital anomaly such as mongolism, arachnoidactyly or a chest deformity of a congenital type. If the patient is cyanosed and clubbed then a congenital heart lesion must be your first consideration if any bruit is present. Often, however, the only valid reason for considering congenital lesions first is the special feature of the bruit. Systolic bruits, which radiate to the left side of the neck and not the right and those which are confined to the left sternal border, are more likely to be due to a congenital than an acquired disease.

With congenital heart lesions a mistake often made is to start by particularizing, mentioning a single and specific congenital lesion, such as atrial septal defect. The far wiser gambit would be to start, 'Sir, this patient has (or probably has, according to the weight of the evidence) a congenital heart lesion such as . . .'. The only congenital lesions that can be diagnosed with certainty clinically are coarctation, patent ductus and, very occasionally, congenital aortic stenosis. It is foolish and conceited to claim that clinically you can differentiate for certainty between atrial and ventricular septal defects or between either and pulmonary stenosis. You are very likely to be proved wrong.

Whether you start with acquired or congenital lesions it is important that you complete your differential diagnosis of all the common causes of either one or the other groups before embarking on a discussion of the alternative group. In other words, never mix up acquired and congenital heart lesions when giving the differential diagnosis, jumping from one group to the other and causing confusion in yourself and the examiner.

If the systolic bruit that you have heard has not got the features expected in the particular condition that you are considering, then the diagnosis should be considered a possibility rather than a probability. For example, if a systolic bruit heard best at the apex is not loud and long then mitral regurgitation is a possibility rather than a probability.

Ninth – A systolic thrill in the region of the apex, especially if confined to that area, is much more likely to be due to a congenital heart lesion than mitral regurgitation.

Tenth – Never start with an aetiology, such as, 'This patient has rheumatic heart disease'. Aetiology should be discussed only after you have considered the certain, the probable and the possible lesions present, because the correctness of the supposed aetiology must depend on the correctness of your diagnosis of the valve lesions.

Eleventh – Remember that hypertension and coronary artery disease, although they are frequently present in the same patient, are two different conditions and may occur independently. Both, together or independently, are common causes of arrhythmias, various types of systolic bruits and cardiac enlargement (although it is often impossible to say whether a cardiac enlargement preceded or was a consequence of a coronary thrombosis).

Twelfth – Never make smart alec or esoteric diagnoses such as ruptured chordae tendineae or ruptured papillary muscle, or mitral prolapse, or whatever happens to be top of the cardiological 'pops' at the moment. To claim that you can make such diagnoses with certainty with your stethoscope is the negation of humility and self-criticism.

Thirteenth – Never use abbreviations such as CCF, JVP, AF, ASD, VSD, PS, MS, AR, etc., because their use is likely to annoy some examiners.

Index